MEDICAL DOCTORS IN HEALTH REFORMS

Also available in the Sociology of Health Professions series

The Allied Health Professions
A Sociological Perspective
Susan Nancarrow and **Alan Borthwick**

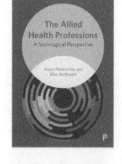

"This excellent book offers a refreshing, sophisticated but eminently readable treatment of theory and inquiry applied to the allied professions."
Anne Rogers, University of Southampton

HB £75.00 ISBN 9781447345367
252 pages March 2021

Support Workers and the Health Professions in International Perspective
The Invisible Providers of Health Care
Edited by **Mike Saks**

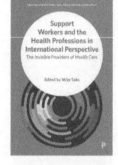

"...a well-written and informative discussion with analysis and description that has the potential to inform current and future workforce planning."
Ian Peate, Gibraltar Health Authority

HB £75.00 ISBN 9781447352105
242 pages July 2020

Professional Health Regulation in the Public Interest
International Perspectives
Edited by **John Martyn Chamberlain**, **Mike Dent** and **Mike Saks**

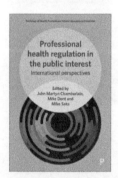

"With enormous variation in the delivery of healthcare, how it is regulated is more important than ever. The authors dissect the differences and enlighten us with forensic ability over a global range." **John Flood**, Griffith University Law School

HB £75.00 ISBN 9781447332268
288 pages June 2018

For more information about the series visit

bristoluniversitypress.co.uk/sociology-of-health-professions

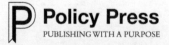

Policy Press
PUBLISHING WITH A PURPOSE

MEDICAL DOCTORS IN HEALTH REFORMS

A Comparative Study of England and Canada

Jean-Louis Denis, Sabrina Germain, Catherine Régis
and Gianluca Veronesi

First published in Great Britain in 2022 by

Policy Press, an imprint of
Bristol University Press
University of Bristol
1–9 Old Park Hill
Bristol
BS2 8BB
UK
t: +44 (0)117 954 5940
e: bup-info@bristol.ac.uk

Details of international sales and distribution partners are available at
policy.bristoluniversitypress.co.uk

© Bristol University Press 2022

British Library Cataloguing in Publication Data
A catalogue record for this book is available from the British Library

ISBN 978-1-4473-5215-0 hardcover
ISBN 978-1-4473-5217-4 ePub
ISBN 978-1-4473-5216-7 ePdf

Cover design by Gareth Davies at Qube Design
Image credit: istock.com/filo
Bristol University Press and Policy Press use environmentally responsible
print partners.
Printed and bound in Great Britain by CPI Group (UK) Ltd, Croydon, CR0 4YY

Contents

List of abbreviations

AI	artificial intelligence
AJMQ	Association des jeunes médecins du Québec [Quebec Association of Young Doctors]
AMQ	Association médicale du Québec [Quebec Medical Association]
APED	assistant president and executive directors
APP	alternate payment plan
BC	British Columbia
BMA	British Medical Association
CCG	Clinical Commissioning Group
CHC	Community Health Clinic
CMA	Canadian Medical Association
CMDP	Council of Medical Doctors, Dentists and Pharmacists
CMP	Conseil pour la protection des malades [Council for the Protection of Patients]
CMPA	Canadian Medical Protective Association
CMQ	Collège des médecins du Québec [College of Physicians of Quebec]
CPSO	College of Physicians and Surgeons of Ontario
CQC	Care Quality Commission
DGH	District General Hospital
DHA	District Health Authority
DRMG	Direction régionale de médecine générale [Regional Directorates of GPs]
EHR	electronic health record
FHN	Family Health Network
FHO	Family Health Organisation
FLQ	Front de libération du Québec [Quebec Liberation Front]
FMG	Family Medicine Group
FMOQ	Fédération des médecins omnipraticiens du Québec [Association of General Practitioners of Quebec]
FMRQ	Fédération des médecins résidents du Québec [Association of Medical Residents of Quebec]
FMSQ	Fédération des médecins spécialistes du Québec [Association of Medical Specialists of Quebec]
GMC	General Medical Council
GMS	General Medical Services
GMSC	General Medical Services Committee
HSO	Health Service Organisation
HSRC	Health Services Restructuring Commission
ICS	Integrated Care Systems

LHIN	Local Health Integration Network
MQRP	Médecins Québécois pour le regime public [Quebec Doctors for a Public System]
MRG	Medical Reform Group
MSIC	Medical Services Insurance Council
NDP	New Democratic Party
NHI	National Health Insurance
NHS	National Health Service
NICE	National Institute for Health and Clinical Excellence
NP	nurse practitioner
NPM	new public management
OHIP	Ontario Health Insurance Plan
OMA	Ontario Medical Association
OMSIP	Ontario Medical Services Insurance Plan
ORAS	Organisation régionale des affaires sociales [Regional Association of Social Affairs]
PC	Progressive Conservative Party of Canada
PCG	Primary Care Group
PCN	Primary Care Network
PCT	Primary Care Trust
PFHS	publicly funded healthcare system
PL	projet de loi [Bill]
PMS	Personal Medical Services
QMA	Québec Medical Association
RAMQ	Régie de l'assurance maladie du Québec [Quebec Health Insurance Board]
RCGP	Royal College of General Practitioners
RHA	Regional Health Authority
SHA	Strategic Health Authority
STP	Sustainability and Transformation Plans

Acknowledgements

This book required a significant amount of research of primary and secondary sources in order to build solid narratives for the Canadian and UK case studies. It would have been impossible to complete this book without help, and we would like to express our gratitude to the following people. We are extremely grateful to Léa Boutrouille, Clara Champagne, François Lamalice and Susan Usher, who were respectively a Bachelors' student in Law at the Université de Montréal, a Master's student in individual study at the Université de Montréal, a Bachelor's student in law at the Université de Montréal, and a Doctoral student in public administration at the École nationale d'administration publique during their work on this book. Their work was rigorous, meticulous and immensely helpful.

We are also in debt to Susan Usher for editing this book. The version you are now reading results from her amazing editing skills that go beyond what anyone can expect from an editor.

Last, but certainly not least, we would like to thank Johanne Préval for being our trusted collaborator on this and so many other projects.

Preface

Health reforms, in theory, aim at creating some form of *systemness*, which includes, on the one hand, a more solid connection between healthcare providers, organisations and professionals and, on the other, the broad policy or systemic goals. The question of medical engagement, leadership and accountability in healthcare system reforms has been an enduring issue in health policy (Baker and Denis, 2011). Medical doctors have played a crucial role in determining the allocation and utilisation of resources in health systems and in shaping capacities to renew policy orientations and models of care (Denis and van Gestel, 2016). This book explores the role of the medical profession in health reforms in two mature welfare states: England and Canada. Both states have a publicly funded healthcare system (PFHS) through taxation. Comparative works on these two systems have already been undertaken by political scientists (Tuohy, 1999, 2012), but less attention has been paid to the specific role of medical doctors in health reforms. The role of the medical profession and the bilateral monopoly between states and the profession have been underlined as a major cause for blockages in health reforms in Canada (Lazar et al, 2013; Tuohy, 2018). In England, the medical profession has been supportive of universality of care, a central element of the National Health Service (NHS); however, during successive waves of reforms medical doctors have fiercely opposed governments' efforts to rationalise the provision of healthcare services, trying to protect egalitarian values at the core of the system and their professional autonomy (Ham, 2009; Klein, 2013). The book investigates the multifaceted and paradoxical situation where a dominant profession – medicine – faces increasing pressures to become an active player and an ally in major policy efforts and system-wide reforms driven by governments.

The conceptual underpinning of this work builds on the contribution of various areas of studies, namely the sociology of professions, studies on professions and organisations and on healthcare law and policy. The analysis documents reformative processes from the inception of two Canadian and the English PFHS, and identifies the role of the medical profession in policy formulation. Our focus is predominantly the role of organised medicine (unions, professional associations and colleges) with their political struggles to promote and advance medical values and interests in a context where governments have attempted to transform healthcare systems. The analysis goes beyond the professional autonomy thesis to understand contemporary manifestations of medical doctors' agency within health reforms. Empirically, the book builds on a socio-historical and institutional narrative (Suddaby and Greenwood, 2009) of healthcare reforms in both England and Canada, and on the role played by the medical profession. Political, organisational, legal and professional dimensions are considered.

The book is structured in six chapters and an epilogue. The Introduction sets out the research objectives and defines the key concepts of healthcare reforms, agency within reforms and the medical profession and government (and State) as the main agents of reform. It looks briefly at the instruments of reform available to government and at the notion of context as an element of analysis. Chapter 1 presents the theoretical framework that underpins the research. Interactions between the two main protagonists – the medical profession and government – take place in a negotiated mediating space shaped by legal and political contexts and coloured by the predispositions of each that evolve in context and through interaction over time to shape reforms. Chapter 2 describes the methodology used to trace the role of medical doctors in healthcare reforms, including the selection of cases in PFHS that enable comparative analysis, data sources and analytical processes.

Chapters 3 and 4 then present the case studies, structured according to a common template. The first section of each chapter provides a detailed case narrative tracing the main periods of reform, with key context events, government reform proposals and the responses and strategies of the medical profession and governments as the reforms unfold. A second section then analyses each of these periods of reform, looking at the drivers and shapers of medical politics, the strategies used by the protagonists, and their implications for medical politics and healthcare reforms.

This common approach to the presentation of each case enables us to provide, in Chapter 5, a comparative analysis, based on our theoretical model, to explain variations and points of convergence across the cases, and to understand how the foundation experience at the start of the PFHS, the approaches taken by government, the institution of medical politics and interactions within the mediated space come together to influence healthcare reforms over time. We conclude the book in Chapter 6 with insights into government's ability to bring about change in healthcare and involve medical doctors in this change.

Editors' overview

This edited text is the fourth in a series entitled the *Sociology of Health Professions: Future International Developments*, published by Policy Press and edited by Mike Saks and Mike Dent, supported by a high-profile international advisory board. The research-based series is focused on giving innovatory sociological insights into the past, present and future development of the health professions. It is mainly oriented towards final year and postgraduate students, academic lecturers/researchers, practitioners and policy-makers. Books included in the series must be resonant with the template for the general Policy Press series on the sociology of the health professions, which aims:

- to inform and stimulate debate about issues in the sociology of health professions;
- to influence policy development and practice in the fields concerned;
- to make a significant contribution to academic thinking in the sociology of health; and
- to produce original national or international work of recognised high quality.

The significance of this book on the role of medical doctors in health reform lies in offering valuable and detailed comparative insights into this subject in England and Canada. As such, Jean-Louis Denis, Sabrina Germain, Catherine Régis and Gianluca Veronesi, as authors of this unique monograph, provide an historical and contemporary analysis that indicates the great, but different, textured influence of these professional groups on health policy in these countries. We therefore again very much welcome this new addition to the Policy Press series on the sociology of the health professions, following *Professional Health Regulation in the Public Interest*, *Support Workers and the Health Professions in International Perspective*, and most recently, *The Allied Health Professions: A Sociological Perspective*, with more fascinating and original commissioned work to come on migration and dentistry in a global context.

Mike Saks and Mike Dent

Introduction: Medical doctors and healthcare reforms

This Introduction defines our research objectives and the key concepts underpinning our inquiry. We look at reforms in contemporary welfare states, which include England and Canada (Denhardt and Denhardt, 2000; Bejerot and Hasselbladh, 2011; Ferlie and McGivern, 2013) and on their implications for the potential roles and manifestations of the agency of medical doctors (Denis et al, 2016).

Setting the scene: reforms in contemporary healthcare systems

The question of healthcare reforms has attracted growing interest among policy analysts and health researchers (Greener, 2009; Ham, 2009; Lazar et al, 2013; Tuohy 2018; Germain, 2019). Reform is a privileged mode of intervention used by liberal democracies to intervene in various policy areas (Rocher, 2008). In their comparative analysis of public management reforms, Pollitt and Bouckaert (2017) define reforms as 'deliberate changes to the structures and processes of a system with the objective of getting them (in some sense) to run better' (Pollitt and Bouckaert, 2017: 2). In the healthcare context, this means improving patient experience, healthcare professionals' satisfaction with work, population health and long-term system viability. Pollitt and Bouckaert's analysis suggests that reform is embedded in a complex web of institutional arrangements and political processes that shape the destiny of reformative ideas and reformers (Marmor and Wendt, 2012; Tuohy, 2018; van Gestel et al, 2018). As suggested by Mechanic and Rochefort (1996), comparable healthcare systems of various nations face similar challenges but their responses vary according to national context and institutions.

Reforms tend to unfold according to sedimentation logic where previous structures, positions and views re-emerge to frame current ambitions and scope for change (Pollitt and Bouckaert, 2017). Timing is central to the process and reinforces the importance of context in shaping the destiny of reforms (van Gestel et al, 2018). In addition, insufficient capacity to resolve persisting issues creates a propensity in some health systems, including in England and Canada, to embark in cyclical reforms (Greener, 2009; Ham, 2009; Forest and Martin, 2018; Germain, 2019). Escalating healthcare costs and technological breakthroughs in drug development, artificial intelligence

(AI) and digital health suggest that systems will face increasing challenges to design, deploy and renew policy instruments. Healthcare reforms, with their trail of destabilisation and reorganisation, are a permanent feature of welfare states (Klein, 2018). Medical doctors are at the forefront of these transformations, with key roles in prescribing medicines, making decisions about the utilisation of resources and facing the impact of these periodic changes.

In their article 'Conceptual frameworks for comparing healthcare politics and policy', Marmor and Wendt (2012) argue that greater attention must be paid to the relation between the structural attributes of healthcare systems, political and institutional dynamics and the outcomes of reforms. Our analysis takes up this challenge, focusing on the role of two specific actors: the medical profession and governments in England and Canada. Persistent problems in publicly funded healthcare systems (PFHS) provide fertile ground for the medical profession to play a greater role in improvement efforts (Baker and Denis, 2011; Spurgeon et al, 2011). In parallel, there is enduring debate around the medical profession's power and capacity to assert its views and interests within health systems, and considerable variation across countries (Laugesen, 2016; Tuohy, 2018). One assumption in our inquiry is that the medical profession maintains an influential role in health policies while simultaneously adapting to changes in context and contingencies. There is therefore a need to better understand empirically how this accommodation transforms and shapes the role of the medical profession in healthcare reforms.

Scholarly work in health policy recognises the growing importance of the quality agenda and the pressure to rationalise use of resources (Klein, 2013; Maynard, 2013; Elshaug et al, 2017; Kleinert and Horton, 2017). Concepts such as learning health systems, value-based care and health equity imply major changes in the way care is delivered and assessed (Porter, 2009; Friedman et al, 2017; Ford-Gilboe et al, 2018). These policy ideas require willing participation, adaptation and a tangible response from the medical profession. The increasingly active role of governments in the direct and indirect steering of health systems also influences the medical profession's involvement in policy change (Greener, 2009). Our analysis of healthcare reforms in England and Canada presents a complex picture of the medical profession's role. While in Canada, medical doctors appear to influence policy changes (Lazar et al, 2013; Tuohy, 2018), in England, Klein (1990, 2018) describes the relation between the State and medical profession as one of mutual dependency and symmetrical frustration.

This research aims to empirically probe the process of managing mutual dependency, symmetrical frustration and differential aspirations between the medical profession and government across various periods of reform in England and in two Canadian provinces: Quebec and Ontario. Reforms are used as revelatory moments in the shaping of relationships between government and the medical profession. While we recognise that other professionals and managers are also influential in shaping the delivery of care, we do not focus on their roles in this analysis, although we do refer to other interest groups when relevant in our inquiry to understand how the relationship between government and the medical profession is influenced by their interferences and voices.

The players: agency in healthcare reforms

The notion of 'agency' is characterised in sociology as polysemic and rather vague. We adopt the definition developed by Emirbayer and Mishe (1998):

> Theoretically, our central contribution is to begin to reconceptualize human agency as a temporally embedded process of social engagement, informed by the past (in its habitual aspect), but also oriented towards the future (as a capacity to imagine alternative possibilities) and towards the present (as a capacity to contextualize past habits and future projects within the contingencies of the moment). The agentic dimension of social action can only be captured in its full complexity, we argue, if it is analytically situated within the flow of time. (Emirbayer and Mishe, 1998: 963)

Through various forms of agency, actors attempt to mediate and transform their relation to context. Medical doctors use their agentic capacities to reposition the profession in regard to the imperatives of reforms. In this process, their agency may have a transformative impact on the content of reforms or on the position and agentic capacities of medical doctors. From a processual perspective, reforms consist of temporary and temporal arrangements resulting from the continuous flow of interpretations and actions in context (Tsoukas and Chia, 2002).

This conception of agency is based on three elements: iteration, projectivity and practical evaluation (Emirbayer and Mishe, 1998: 970). *Iteration* refers to the selective reactivation of past experiences and practices. Engrained conceptions of professionalism and the memory of past conflictual or harmonious relations will shape the conduct of medical doctors and their reaction to reforms. The *projective* element refers to the creative ability to anticipate and conceive of possibilities for the future. An example would be the engagement of medical doctors in prospective thinking to envision the future of medicine and the profession's role in healthcare systems. The *practical-evaluative* element consists in an agent's ability to make practical and normative judgements about various options in an immediate context (the

3

present) characterised by contingencies, dilemmas and opportunities. An example would be the assessment made by medical doctors of the potential and limitations of a reform in primary care.

In empirical situations, these three elements of agency combine in various unexpected ways. Our inquiry focuses on how medical doctors and governments invest these three elements of agency in healthcare reforms. Agency is conceived as a situated practice where past experiences, desirable futures and immediate contingencies combine and shape reactions to reform.

The medical profession as an agent of reform

The medical profession can be defined as:

> An occupation whose core element is work based upon the mastery of a complex body of knowledge and skills. It is a vocation in which knowledge of some department of science or learning or the practice of an art founded upon it is used in the service of others. Its members are governed by codes of ethics and profess a commitment to competence, integrity and morality, altruism, and the promotion of the public good within their domain. These commitments form the basis of a social contract between a profession and society, which in return grants the profession a monopoly over the use of its knowledge base, the right to considerable autonomy in practice and the privilege of self-regulation. Professions and their members are accountable to those served and to society. (Cruess et al, 2004: 75)

This definition stresses 'disinterestedness' as one of the fundamental functionalist criteria of 'professions' (Torstendahl, 2005). According to this definition of agency and this essentialist view of professions, medical doctors engage in and react to healthcare reforms according to their conceptions of professional autonomy and professionalism. A complex set of practical and normative considerations structures their interpretation of healthcare reforms.

Our analysis focuses on the collective manifestation of medical doctors' agency in healthcare reforms: the actions and reactions of groups or individuals as representatives of organised segments of the profession, such as professional associations, militant groups of medical doctors, professional unions and professional elites of all sorts. We look at the ability of a collective agent to engage in voluntary and independent actions within the constraints of prevailing social structures and arrangements (Campbell, 2009). The participation of medical doctors in reforms is based on complex patterns of involvement in context.

Governments or states as agents of reform

The term 'reformer' is used here to refer to entities that have the authority and the legitimacy to develop and implement policies in order to act on the structure, functioning, performance and viability of PFHS. The main entity of interest in our analysis is government, although we recognise that reformers can also be located in more diffuse networks outside formal organisations (Tuohy, 2012). We consider governments as the main driver in setting the stage for reforms through policy development and using legal instruments. In this research, government forms the other side of the agentic force field that shapes healthcare reforms.

The distinction between State and government needs to be underlined. While the notions of State and government are closely associated, they are not synonymous (Jensen, 2008). The former is predominantly seen as an abstraction, with the latter its concrete application. The terms are not interchangeable and unjustified replacement of the term 'State' by 'government' in certain propositions undermines the intended meaning (Barry, 1989: 67).

In political theory, the State is described by philosopher Joseph Raz as the 'political organization of a society', and government as the 'agent through which it acts' (Raz, 1986: 70). As Robert Crane puts it, the 'State is now conceived as an abstraction, something over and above its physical members' (Crane, 1907: 39), and thus pursues higher values than those of ordinary individuals (Barry, 1989: 58, note 2). German legal scholars in the 19th century further distinguish the State from its sovereignty and the machinery it uses to execute its will (that is, government) (Crane, 1907: 40, note 4). More recent scholars insist that the concept of State should be strictly *opposed* to the personal power held by individuals at the head of the State to avoid compromising a comprehensive concept of State as the institutionalisation of power (Nettl, 1968).

In analysis fairly consistent with the definition given by sociologist Max Weber (Gerth and Wright Mills, 1948: 78), British academic Bob Jessop identifies the key components of the State: a state territory (or determined geographical boundaries), a state apparatus that enables decision-making, and a state population (Jessop, 2011: 239–41). Other features of the State include the public nature of its rules and the centralisation of its authority and coercive power (Robertson, 2002: 211).

The notion of government refers to public institutions' practical functioning, policy-making authority and ability to implement decisions (Jensen, 2008, note 1). This notion embodies the institutions that possess the executive authority of a collectivity (Robertson, 2002, note 10). In modern societies, the executive function is fulfilled by the government and crown corporations, which have distinct legal personalities and together, exercise regulatory, discretionary and administrative powers.

In this book, we are most interested in the notion of 'government' as it embeds a form of agency in State actors that materialises during the reform process. Governments undertake reform programmes, design laws and provide resources for the implementation of reforms. They exercise the agentic capacity that makes reforms possible. Governments also operate and interact with the medical profession, within the mediated space of reforms. That said, when we specifically refer to the more neutral and abstract form of State action, we use the word 'State'.

Policy instruments and the agency of governments in healthcare reforms

One of the key features of contemporary polity is the development and reliance on a diverse set of policy instruments. As proposed by Salamon (2002: 19), policy instruments are 'an identifiable method through which collective action is structured to address a public problem'. The growing interest in policy instruments (Hood, 1983; Linder and Peters, 1989; Schneider and Ingram, 1990; Doern and Phidd, 1992; Salamon, 2002) is symptomatic of changes in the way governments attempt to exert influence in various policy areas (Lascoumes and Le Galès, 2007). Reforms incorporate a complex and diversified set of policy instruments in an attempt to translate ideas and objectives into substantive changes. The framework developed by Schneider and Ingram (1990) sees governments rely on different tools to achieve reforms: authority tools, incentive tools, capacity tools, symbolic and horatory tools, and learning tools.

Authority tools refer to laws and regulations and are based on the assumption that the targets are inclined to obey or conform to them. This could be a law that obliges medical doctors to work in rural areas for a certain number of years after graduation. *Incentive tools* consist of tangible payoffs to induce compliance. An incentive may be positive, such as a bonus paid to perform preventive screening, or negative, such as a decrease in annual income if targets are not met. *Capacity tools* refer to resources that enable agents to perform particular tasks or achieve policy goals. Training programmes for quality improvement are one example. *Symbolic and horatory tools* appeal to values and beliefs to induce compliance with policy goals. Appealing to professionals' sense of public duty to avoid waste in the health system is a good example. Reformers can also rely on *learning tools* to promote broadly defined policy goals such as care and service integration. Learning tools reflect that governments are not always clear on what strategy might solve a collective problem, and rely on knowledgeable actors to experiment, evaluate and share experiences. In the context of this study, we expect that governments will use a variety of policy instruments and tools across periods of reform to effect change.

Distal and proximal context variables

As highlighted earlier, this book recognises the vital importance of context when analysing how reforms emerge and unfold. It also brings out the complexity and richness of context as an element of analysis, beyond what is acknowledged in the existing literature, which does not always identify political, legal and organisational factors that influence the process of healthcare reforms. We distinguish elements of context through distal and proximal variables. *Distal variables* relate to the political, legal and institutional landscapes of a given jurisdiction that are not directly associated with a given healthcare reform. In other words, they are relevant and ubiquitous, yet somewhat independent of the specific reform under investigation. The distal variables are antecedents and *ex-ante* components of law and politics, such as the constitutional division of legislative powers between different levels of government, or fundamental rights. Distal context variables ultimately impact on how governments think about reforms and reflect secular trends or potential evolutions (*in abstracto*). *Proximal variables* exist *in situ*, within the system of relationships and contingencies associated with a specific reform in the healthcare policy arena. Proximal context is conceived as the sum of endogeneity and learning triggered by a healthcare reform, as well as the interpretation and appropriation of elements of the distal context that are consequential for a given reform. Specific financial constraints or a government's ideological position are two examples. Empirically, distal and proximal dimensions of context combine and overlap to frame actors' predispositions and manifestations of agency in healthcare reforms.

Agency in healthcare reforms

This Introduction defines some of the key constructs used in our inquiry and delineates its boundaries as the dual agency of – and mutual dependency between – the medical profession and government in the becoming of healthcare reforms. Governments accommodate and capitalise on their mutual dependency with the medical profession using diverse sets of policy instruments and tools; these influence the ability of agents to arrive at political agreements in reforms. The participation and reaction of the medical profession to reforms will be contingent on the specific policy instruments or tools associated with the reformative template, on a wide set of proximal and distal contextual factors, and on the immediate practicality of certain options and future aspirations.

1

Theoretical framework

This chapter presents the conceptual framework underpinning our research. It looks at elements of the legal and political context that influence the role of medical doctors in healthcare reforms. It then analyses scholarly work on the sociology of professions and the interface between professions and organisations in order to better understand the predispositions of medical doctors in the context of reforms. The chapter closes with a presentation of the theoretical model that guides our empirical inquiry.

Agency in context: legal and political dimensions

Social scientists have long been interested in the study of change in institutions (Pettigrew et al, 2001), which requires attention to the intricacies of context (political, economic and legal), history and process that impact on change (Langley et al, 2013). Context is thus considered an environment in which agency and change co-evolve as a response to situational or conjectural opportunities and limitations (Johns, 2006). Norms and rules within a given context limit or encourage the expression of human agency. For example, national political and legal institutions (Immergut, 1990), such as courts with judicial power, provide an overarching context that shapes the negotiating space where governments and medical doctors engage in reforms.

In this first section we focus on specific components of the legal and political context that condition the space in which governments and professions interact in healthcare reforms. Legal and political elements associated with this context operate alongside secular trends such as changing demographics, economic conditions and technological and epidemiological shifts to impact the healthcare system's ability to meet population needs.

Law as a context for the expression of agency in healthcare reforms

Law is part of the distal and proximal context that influences opportunities for agency in healthcare reforms. The influence is twofold. First, law plays an overarching role in framing the agentic capacities of governments and medical doctors. While the notion of agency refers to the capacity of actors or entities to act on a situation and demonstrate free will, the agentic capacities of governments and the medical profession are conditioned by legal constraints and imperatives. As a distal consideration, law sometimes affects *ex-ante* options for healthcare reforms, for instance by limiting the policy options available to governments wishing to coerce medical doctors into acting a certain way or modifying rules around access to care. In *de jure* societies like England and Canada, the rule of law precludes arbitrary modes of governance, since the actions of the executive branch are conducted in accordance with the law and with the highest enforceable norm, which, in Canada, is the Constitution (*Reference re Secession of Québec*, 1998, para 72[1]) and in England, the laws of Parliament that form a non-codified constitution (Barnett, 2020: 121). Courts also play an instrumental role in the enforcement of these norms. Constitutions encase systems of governance that flesh out the structure, powers and duties of government, as well as the fundamental rights conferred on citizens, including medical doctors (Boylan-Kemp, 2008: 1). In Canada these rights are defined by the Canadian Charter of Rights and Freedoms[2], whereas in England they are defined by statutes and quasi-constitutional laws that significantly affect fundamental rights and duties and relations between citizens (Samuels, 2018: 1). In order to produce enforceable laws, governments must abide by their constitutional duties.

Second, law structures government's ability to propose legal norms and use coercive instruments instead of capacity tools to enforce policy. As an endogenic component of health systems, law also influences how healthcare reforms unfold. The relationship between medical doctors and governments, especially during reforms, influences whether and how the law is mobilised. For instance, a government could choose to deal with deadlocked negotiations by introducing a special law to implement its desired policy and force the medical profession to comply. However, as an element of the proximal context, the law also imposes boundaries within which the government can operate. In Québec, the court stated on different occasions that government must act according to its legislation and avoid contradictory behaviours. Two examples help explain this logic: (1) if the government makes abortion a publicly funded service, it then has a duty to react when the public system fails to provide adequate access to abortion (*Association pour l'accès à l'avortement c. Québec*, 2006 QCCS 4694, [2006] RJQ 1938t); and (2) if the government limits access to private insurance to protect the integrity of the publicly funded healthcare system, it must ensure that public healthcare services are provided in accordance with fundamental rights to life and security (and therefore ensure timely access) (*Chaoulli vs Québec* (Attorney General), 2005 SCC 35). In England, legal instruments also impose duties on the government with regard to healthcare: the Secretary of State is obliged to 'provide comprehensive health services' in accordance with the boundaries set by the Health and Social Care Act 2012 (Article 1).

While legal tools can help governments assert power during the reform process, they provide more limited opportunity to exercise authority over the regular provision of healthcare. The extent to which legal instruments provide leverage during healthcare reforms depends on the government's depth of reform and leadership style (collaborative or authoritative). Heavy reliance on legal tools (laws, regulations, enforcement mechanisms) to impose policies may impact medical doctors' willingness to work towards the reform's objectives. It also diverges from the recent tendency to diversify the set of policy instruments used in reforms (we come back to this point later).

Instrumental authoritative leadership has higher compliance costs, requiring more public resources (financial and human) to monitor and enforce. Making laws involves multiple legislative steps and a variety of actors, while enforcement requires financing institutions and actors such as judges, public inspectors and police officers. This type of leadership also contradicts the collaborative endeavour at the core of PFHS. The many relational and institutional interdependencies that characterise healthcare systems (Marcus et al, 2011) require that all actors, including medical doctors and governments, work together towards achieving social and clinical goals.

Politics as an enabling and constraining context for healthcare reforms

This section briefly examines some of the broader social forces that favour a closer relationship between governments and the medical profession. First, some authors in the sociology of professions distinguish between public sector professions, private sector professions and more liberal professions (Ackroyd, 2016). These different professions have populated public services in a context of State expansion since the Second World War. Public sector professions (*medical doctors* in PFHS, for example) are *de facto* more exposed to government demands than professions such as accountants or lawyers. Relations between public sector professions and government are crucial to the profession's status, role and evolution. Public sector professions embark in *regulatory bargains* (Macdonald, 1995; Ackroyd, 2016) with government to secure and protect their conditions of practice (1995). The objective is to secure a '*social contract*' with the State that will guarantee status, privileges and autonomy to a given profession in exchange for service responsibilities.

In line with a neo-Weberian approach to professions, public sector professionalism is conceived both as an ethos – dedication to providing a service that is valued by the State as a public good – and a status, bestowing autonomy, self-regulation and self-jurisdiction on an occupational group; both are relatively immune to market forces (Saks, 2010). Public sector professionals can be salaried employees of governments or publicly owned organisations, or they can act independently, with their services covered by public funding. In both instances, public sector professionals such as medical doctors work under different conditions than professions driven by a private sector ethos (that is, accountants and lawyers in private firms) (Greenwood and Suddaby, 2006; Morris et al, 2010). Saks and colleagues (Saks, 2016; Saks and Adams, 2019) have explored, from a neo-Weberian perspective, the historical struggle of the medical profession to secure occupational closure and privileges in the labour market. Governments have responded positively to these pressures and demands from the medical profession and conferred on medical doctors a privileged position in the labour market. This raises the question of whether professional groups have subordinated their own interests to the wider public interest in carrying out their work (Saks, 1995).

Some public sector professions have more bargaining power with government than others (think of medical doctors vs teachers, for example). Bargaining dynamics are an important factor in the emergence and consolidation of an organised (or unionised) profession defending and securing their vision, interests and occupational niche. Depending on the jurisdiction, professions will be more or less organised to engage in and influence negotiations with government regarding their role, status and autonomy. For example, there are differences between the role in health policy played by the British Medical Association (BMA), the Canadian Medical Association (CMA), and the medical doctors' unions in each Canadian province. Our analysis focuses on how relations between the medical profession and government influence health reforms and, more broadly, health policies within PFHS. In this regard, we take as a starting point the State's endorsement of the medical profession's status and the need for the profession to affirm and defend its interests during various periods of health reforms (Saks, 2010, 2016). We take stock of the theoretical and empirical insights gained from the neo-Weberian analysis of professions, and explore the medical profession's ability to capitalise on its occupational niche and status to voice and promote its views on health reforms and protect its interests.

Reforms can be seen as a deliberate attempt by government to renegotiate the regulatory bargain with public sector professions (Ackroyd et al, 1989). This contract, or bargaining process, is crucial to manage the interdependence between profession and State, and is thus considered a contingent political process where the meaning of changes is contested (Bevir et al, 2003).

Rethinking agency through the governmentalisation of the State, authors like Bevir (2013), Waring and Bevir (2017) and Ferlie and colleagues (2008) propose the concept of 'narratives' to describe the broad approaches or steering patterns adopted by governments to intervene in policy areas. The analysis of professions, inspired by a Foucauldian perspective on governmentality (Bevir, 2011; Ferlie and McGivern, 2013), suggests that the profession is increasingly embedded in the regulatory enterprise of contemporary States through the activation and contestation of narratives of reform. Narratives are not pure analytical frameworks aiming at comprehension (in the Weberian sense), but rather, 'mix technical and also political and normative elements'

(Ferlie et al, 2008: 334). These narratives are defined in various ways. Pollitt and Bouckaert (2017), for example, rely on the following classification: new public management (NPM), network governance and new Weberian state. Our analysis is less concerned with how the specificities of each narrative shape the role of professions in reforms than with the importance of States and governments as forces – the concept of *steering patterns* – that orient the development of professions and their roles.

Narratives (or *steering patterns*), such as the adoption of evidence-based decision-making or behavioural economics, are prominent in contemporary healthcare reforms. They are associated with the proliferation of new and often indirect policy instruments that embody an implicit theory of power-knowledge (Lascoumes and Le Galès, 2004, 2010). Knowledge and mentalities – that is, the way individuals and groups frame the definition of and solutions to public problems – are constitutive of these technologies of power (Bevir, 2013). Consensual politics are a core feature of this expanding role of policy instruments in contemporary regimes of governmentality (Lascoumes and Le Galès, 2004). Reliance on a new set of policy instruments implies the emergence of a governmentality regime that acts through an agent's freedom (Martin and Waring, 2018). From a governmentality perspective, there is place for agency, counter-conduct and eventually co-development of reforms (Bevir, 2010). Policy instruments act as mediators in the relationship between government and profession (in formal terms, the governed).

This 'governmentalisation' of the State has parallels with the idea of the regulatory State in political science (Pildes and Sunstein, 1995; Rose et al, 2006; Rose and Miller, 2010; Power, 2011). The notion of the regulatory state captures the fact that modern States face complex new challenges and respond by renovating their policy instruments and capacities. The specificities and salience of health politics (Carpenter, 2012) in contemporary societies stimulates and somewhat exacerbates initiatives to transform and adapt regulations and use regulatory power differently. Healthcare reform is conceived as a symptom of the progressive enrolment of professionals, and more specifically, medical doctors, in a larger sphere of politics and cultural change where institutions aspire to create and stabilise multiple systems of actors (Meyer, 2010).

Our assumption is that medical doctors have been progressively integrated into the regulatory and normalisation apparatus of government. Their expertise is incorporated into a political, legal and cultural project that transcends their immediate self-interest, claims and aspirations. Changes in knowledge, task complexity, technologies and expectations induce demand for reform, which then opens up new regulatory capacities and possibilities promoted by governments. This development is not just the result of government's subjectivation or disciplinary power, but is also a manifestation of the agentic capacities of medical doctors (Martin and Waring, 2018). There is thus an apparent convergence between Freidson's (1985) hypothesis of professional re-stratification, which implies the emergence of new professional elites within the medical profession (such as quality and safety directors), and the Foucauldian perspective on governmentality where actors become active developers of control and regulation mechanisms in a given field.

Context and reforms

Considered as elements of the distal context, the impact of these legal and political factors on healthcare reforms is likely to be mediated by the position and influence of agents within the healthcare system and by interactions between these agents. The distal context may be especially important when controversies around elements of reform give rise to legitimate recourse to law to assert positions or shape the *modus operandi* of political forces in public domains. The law and legal institutions, such as the courts, may also trigger reforms or policy shifts if citizens, medical doctors or other healthcare professionals oppose current policies or practices in healthcare systems. The emergence of the regulatory State and the governmentalisation of politics may have deep and enduring effects on the manifestation of various stakeholders' agency in reforms. Growing interdependence between profession and State, at least with public sector professions, and the ability to rely on safeguards and the rule of law are two broad forces that shape our conceptual viewpoint on healthcare reforms. Assessing these forces in the context of a specific reform is of empirical importance.

Sociological and organisational perspectives on the role of medical doctors in healthcare reforms

This section turns to the endogeneity of healthcare reforms, where different drivers of change and learning take shape. It explores the evolving interface between professions and organisations as a space where tensions, authority and accommodation co-exist. We see multiple factors in healthcare pushing to further integrate the medical profession within organised settings and networks. This institutional change transforms professions and organisations, and suggests that reformative forces build on these evolutionary trends.

Status and roles of professions

Here we look at various perspectives and arguments from the sociology of professions. The purpose is not to systematically and exhaustively review the scholarship in these fields (for this, we recommend recent reviews of the sociology of medicine and sociology within medicine – see Hafferty and Castellani, 2011 – and reviews of recent developments in the sociology of professions – Adams, 2015; Suddaby and Muzio, 2015; Saks, 2016), but rather to gain analytical traction on the problem of medical doctors' involvement and agency in reforms. To this end, we explore various representations of the profession, identify challenges faced in securing occupational status and niche, and describe professional responses to changing contexts and situations.

The sociology of professions represents a rich body of work based on various intellectual traditions and influenced by the national context in which studies of professions are performed (Adams, 2015). In their review of the sociology *of* medicine and sociology *in* medicine, Hafferty and Castellani (2011) suggest that current trends towards a renewal of professionalism within the medical profession (Cruess et al, 2000; Evetts, 2013; Dingwall, 2016) have focused attention on the role played by exogenous factors (such as secular economic and demographic trends, shifting political ideologies and new societal expectations) in the evolution of contemporary medicine. An understanding of how professional motives combine with these exogenous factors appears crucial to fully comprehend the role of medical doctors in reforms.

The essentialist or taxonomic approach to the study of professions

Early sociological contributions in the field attempt to define a set of attributes or traits that distinguish a profession from other work roles or occupational categories (Saks, 2010). This *essentialist* or *taxonomic* view is closely associated with a functionalist perspective according to which professions play an indispensable role in society and preserve social order (Mauss and Durkheim, 1937; Parsons, 1939; Adams, 2015). The main idea is that professions develop to respond to specific functional needs in society (achieving equilibrium, responding to the risk of political instability associated with modernisation, evaluating rationality or scientific progress) (Drazin, 1990; Macdonald, 1995).

From a functionalist perspective, the status and role of the medical profession are well aligned with societal and organisational expectations (Schneyer, 2013). In periods of destabilisation or social transformation, reforms aim to restore this alignment. Using various levers (legislation, incentives, and so on), society intervenes to realign the medical profession with factors that signal a need for change and adaptation (Crompton, 1990). According to this perspective, organisations can be perceived as institutions that exist as a means for professions to render services, enabling professionals to enact their knowledge and specialised expertise while being driven by a sense of altruism and acting as public trustees. Organisations are the spaces where professionals are given the opportunity to look after the welfare of the individual (Marshall, 1939), pursue public safety and enhance service quality. The hospital is perceived as the doctor's workshop (Kitchener et al, 2005) and is characterised as a professional bureaucracy (Mintzberg, 1979). Competition is a barrier for professionals as it limits their material security, altruistic orientation and public service ethos (Parsons, 1954); hence, healthcare organisations need to be protected from market forces to achieve their objectives.

However, while organisations can be seen as providing support to professions, they may also conflict with professional aspirations. The tension between organisational and professional spheres originates in the incompatibility (apparent or real) between professional values of autonomy, commitment to service and expert knowledge, and the organisation's traditional bureaucratic values of control, discipline and compliance with rules (Gouldner, 1957, 1958; Blau and Scott, 1962; Gunz and Gunz, 2006). Professional behaviour is influenced by training and specialised knowledge, while bureaucratic norms emphasise organisational authority (Gouldner, 1957; Raelin, 1986). From an essentialist viewpoint, medical doctors' reactions to reforms are also influenced by the singularity of the relationship between profession and organisation.

The profession as an achievement: a processual approach to the study of professions

Moving from an essentialist approach to a socio-historical or critical approach reveals the fragility and complexity of the professional project. Professionals have not always enjoyed a dominant position in their field as the essentialist approach assumes. The existence of tensions between various institutional logics (for example, professional and managerial logics) underlines the limitations of the essentialist approach. The question of how the development, mobilisation and reproduction of expert knowledge coincides with the recognition of professional status and power in society is a predominant theme in the sociology of professions (Larson, 1979; Freidson, 1988; McKinlay and Marceau, 2002). This processual view (Pettigrew, 1992; Langley et al, 2013) considers professions as an achievement and an aspiration.

This approach to the study of professions incorporates a sociological view of power (as a resource) with regard to the relationship between professions, societies and organisations. Rooted in Weberian sociology and a critical approach to the role of professions in society, 'professional groups are directly or indirectly conceptualized in terms of exclusionary social closure in the marketplace, sanctioned by the state' (Saks, 2010: 887). The role of the government is, therefore, crucial in credentialing and providing control over segments of practice and ultimately in making professional monopoly possible (Brint, 1993; Freidson, 1988; Abbott, 2005). The notion of labour market shelter or societal closure is employed to suggest that professionals struggle for a very specific occupational status immune (to various degrees) from market pressure and external interference (Paradeise, 1988; Leicht and Fennell, 1997). This is the essence of a neo-Weberian approach to professions (Saks, 2010). Health reforms that appear to challenge the integrity of such an occupational niche by imposing new external controls, and in some cases direct market control, will face resistance and counter-reactions from the medical profession. Our inquiry focuses on the tensions and accommodations between the perceived need for governments' intervention to regulate medical practice and behaviours using reforms, and the medical profession's aspirations to self-regulate. Thus, professionals will engage in institutional work to maintain control over their occupational niche (Muzio et al, 2013), including use of social mechanisms such as demonstration of commitment, strong sense of identity and solidarity among members of the profession (Freidson, 1988; Brint, 1993). However, countervailing powers are at play to act on and transform professions and professional work (Light, 1995), meaning that there is no absolute guarantee that the profession can generate and activate power circuits and resources to sustain its specific occupational status (Clegg, 1989).

Interestingly, some authors who depart from essentialist or taxonomic approaches highlight the benefits of the anomalous status and position of professions in the labour market (Paradeise, 1988). What is implied here is that professions and protected occupational shelters are related to the pursuit of values such as safeguarding citizens and service users from growing interference by hierarchical controls and market competition. The profession is seen as an institutional logic that combats forces of alienation or rationalisation (Freidson, 2001). While the medical profession, like other professions, may occasionally need to fight to maintain ground they have conquered in terms of status, privileges and autonomy in the labour market (Larson, 1979; Mckinlay and Arches, 1985), this struggle develops around both the preservation of professional interests and the safeguarding and promotion of societal ideals (Adler et al 2008, 2015). These two views often conflate in exchanges between State, government and the medical profession, and are considered in our analysis. The dividing line between professional and public interest can be difficult to assess empirically. Resistance to reformative propositions on the part of the profession also reveals a struggle for the preservation of a professional ethos to the benefit of societies. Or it could represent an attempt to protect professional interests regardless of more general public interests.

From this viewpoint, organisations represent the space where professions exercise their power and mobilise knowledge to control expert work; they are instruments through which professions accumulate social and financial rewards. Organisations are controlled by a restricted group of professional elites to limit outsiders' access to privileges and benefits (Parkin, 1979; Freidson, 1994) and protect the professional domain from outside forces, especially managerial encroachments (Noordegraaf, 2015). However, the integration of professionals into formal organisations reveals the challenges of maintaining a privileged occupational niche. Professionals are unlikely 'to fit well within formal organisations' (Gunz and Gunz, 2006: 259) due to conflicts between professional autonomy and organisational control (Noordegraaf, 2011; Suddaby and Muzio, 2015). Autonomy and status are limited when exercised within organisational boundaries (Wilensky, 1964; Etzioni, 1969; Evetts, 2004).

Reforms that attempt to change the hierarchy of professional and organisational norms and expectations culminate in resistance or open opposition from professionals. The status of professions – no longer a given – results from the day-to-day efforts of professionals to protect and expand occupational control over their work and the power to self-organise (Johnson, 1972; Freidson, 1988, 1994; Reed, 1996). Accounts of professionalism frequently focus on the existence of an inherent conflict in the relationship between professions and organisations (Cooper and Robson, 2006; Suddaby et al, 2007; Muzio and Kirkpatrick, 2011).

Theories of professions based on Marxian ideas (a conflict sociology approach; see Collins and Sanderson, 2015) also place the notion of asymmetric power relations and the pursuit of self-interest at the core of their analysis, with consequences for individual and collective professional behaviour. Marxian accounts suggest that social and economic demands within organisations represent increasing challenges to professional autonomy (Saks, 2012), legitimising bureaucratic control (Johnson, 1972). Processes of routinisation, rationalisation and commodification through de-skilling lead to de-professionalisation (Haug, 1972, 1988; Reed and Evans, 1987) and the proletarianisation of professionals (Oppenheimer, 1972; McKinlay and Arches, 1985; Elston, 2002; Sehested, 2002; Johnson et al, 1995; Bejerot and Hasselbladh, 2011). Economic forces and technological advancements are influential forms of occupational control and underline the fragility of professions in the face of labour market transformations (see, for example, Braverman Labour Process Theory, 1974; Littler, 1990), culminating in the subjugation of professional work (Freidson, 1983; Hafferty and Light, 1995; Leicht and Fennell, 1997).

This constellation of factors and forces provides fertile ground to contest the legitimacy and preservation of control over an occupational niche, and is accompanied by pressures to reframe the meaning and manifestation of professional autonomy. Occupational niches and market shelters have to be defended against these powerful forces (Brock et al, 2013), and professionals and professions necessarily face pressure to change. To what extent these forces have significantly transformed the power and status of the medical profession is an empirical question, and reforms can be interpreted as a compact between opposing forces. Medical doctors cannot avoid the pressure for change and, consequently, become more active in shaping the trajectory of healthcare reforms.

Institutional context and the agentic capacities of professionals

According to Suddaby and Muzio (2015), organisational scholars' interest in professions dates back to studies in the early 1960s looking at how professionals structured their work within large bureaucratic organisations such as hospitals, which were growing in size and number of professionals (Montagna, 1968; Buchanan, 1974; Larson, 1977). Understanding the process of reconciling professional autonomy and bureaucratic imperatives is at the heart of an institutional approach to change in professional organisations.

Unlike the power lens, this approach looks at professions as institutions, in the sense that they 'represent distinctive and identifiable structures of knowledge, expertise, work and labour markets, with distinct norms, practices, ideologies and organizational forms' (Leicht, 2005: 604). Broad transformations in the institutional context of professionalism lead to a reconfiguration and relocation of professional activity within the boundaries of increasingly large and complex organisations (Dacin et al, 2002; Hinings, 2005; Brock et al, 2007; Leicht and Fennell, 2008). As actors highly involved in processes of institutional change, professions create new jurisdictions for particular expertise (Abbott, 1988), generate new organisational forms such as multi-hospital integrated healthcare systems (Scott et al, 2000), and control access and career advancements in the field (Siebert et al, 2016). Essentially, neo-institutional theory accounts for the self-interest of the profession (power lens) as well as the professional pursuit of public interest (functionalist lens). The institutional lens more fully takes into account the agentic and societal roles of professions, as it incorporates the idea that professions shape but are also shaped by the institutional environment (Suddaby and Muzio, 2015). Healthcare reforms can be considered a plausible vehicle to transform and simultaneously reaffirm the roles, status and values of the medical profession. Professions represent an achievement that is constantly debated and redefined as they adapt and respond to changes and expectations that emanate from distal and proximal changes and forces.

Professionals are thus considered key agents of social change thanks to their prominent and powerful position in the field (DiMaggio and Powell, 1983; Denis et al, 2016). Professionalisation projects fundamentally embed endogenous projects of institutionalisation (Reed, 1996; Hwang and Powell, 2005; Scott, 2008; Suddaby and Viale, 2011) and represent endogenous processes of institutional change, reconfiguring institutions as well as fields.

Resistance to or acceptance of change is affected by how power is enacted (DiMaggio and Powell, 1991; Scott et al, 2000; McNulty and Ferlie, 2002; Ferlie et al, 2005). As 'lords of the dance' (Scott, 2008), professions have a predominant role in creating and shaping institutions, playing a crucial part in the organisation and re-ordering of social life. Medical doctors not only react or accommodate, but also shape reforms, including through institutional work within healthcare organisations.

Processes of change and accommodation within professions and organisational fields

In parallel with advancements in institutional theory, other organisational scholars embrace a different understanding of the changes affecting professionalism (Noordegraaf, 2013, 2015). They suggest that the norm for professionals is to operate in (normally) well-organised contexts congruent with the organisation of professional practice (Denis et al, 2013). Rather than needing protection from organisational forces, professionalism is incorporated within organisational principles and structures, and this embeddedness allows professionals to benefit from organisational assets to achieve professional virtuosity. Along these lines, Noordegraaf (2011) associates the emergence of 'organised professionalism' with the evolving relationship between external changes, organisational contexts and professional work. Thus, this perspective moves beyond arguments based strictly on conflicting accounts of professionals in organisations and looks at how professionals and organisations can co-exist and work in synergy to achieve shared or convergent goals (see, for example, Pollitt, 1993; Harrison and Pollitt, 1994; Clarke and Stewart, 1997; Abramovitz, 2005; Morrell, 2006) as well as cope with market pressures (De Bruijn, 2010).

Broad institutional, social and societal forces – changing work preferences, multifaceted and increasingly complex problems, and higher levels of risk – impact on professionals in tangible ways. They not only radically reconfigure professional work, but also question the nature of professional (self-)control and render boundaries between professional work and organisational practices more fluid (Suddaby et al, 2009; Evetts, 2011; Noordegraaf, 2013). Organisational environments are no longer seen as constraints on the exercise of professional work, and the relationship between professions and organisations appears less transactional (Adler et al, 2008; Adler and Kwon, 2013). Professional regulation – standards and rules – that was previously developed and maintained autonomously by professionals – is now increasingly generated within organisations (Cooper and Robson, 2006). This leads to a form of hybridisation of professionalism, which requires balancing 'opposite' principles such as autonomy and control with quality and efficiency (McGivern et al, 2015; Noordegraaf, 2015). The new model of professionalism moves past 'uneasy' hybridisation (Harrison, 1993) to incorporate organising as a normal part of professional work: 'organising is part of the job' (Noordegraaf, 2015: 16). Again, the fluidity of these changes is a question to be explored empirically in the context of specific jurisdictions and reforms.

Importantly, Nordegraaf (2015) stresses that professionalism is also reshaped outside organisational boundaries, embedded in the selection of professionals, their education, training and socialisation. New obligations arising from external influences such as work and demographic shifts, complexity of cases, emergence of new types of risk and legitimacy in the public eye have led professional associations to design new principles, models and approaches for the reorganisation of professional work (Noordegraaf, 2011). Shifts in professional organising arise from accepting (rather than opposing; see Larson, 1977; Freidson, 1985) contemporary expectations for professional practice and standards of behaviour (Denis et al, 2016).

Organisations, professions and reforms

In the context of healthcare reforms, advances in organisational and institutional analysis suggest that the medical profession may play a very different role from the one expected within a power and conflict view of professionalism. There is an understanding that exogenous pressures demand that the profession will be willing to consider a multiplicity of interests, needs and principles. Professional and public interests may be less antagonistic or get redefined and mixed (realigned) in the process of reforms. The default position of the profession is no longer opposed to alternative logics of organising. In the neo-institutional perspective, the profession itself can become an agent of change in the sense of not only accepting, but also meaningfully pursuing, efforts to meet broader societal expectations. Furthermore, the profession need not be 'coerced' into accepting modifications to its status and privileges, but may actively negotiate changes with the understanding that a form of compromise has to be achieved for reforms to be adopted. Modifications in the fundamental concept of professionalism are partly internalised, and external demands and pressures are, to some extent, embraced as professional issues. The mosaic of forces that shape reforms is complex, and influence is conditioned by how agents interpret evolving societal expectations and how they capitalise on them by manifesting agency. Power and conflict perspectives on professions, organisations and societies provide a productive lens to understand the plausibility of the role of professionals as agents of institutional change. In the next section, we propose an integrated theoretical framework to guide our empirical analysis of the role of medical doctors in healthcare reforms in England and Canada.

Figure 1.1: The role of medical doctors in healthcare reforms

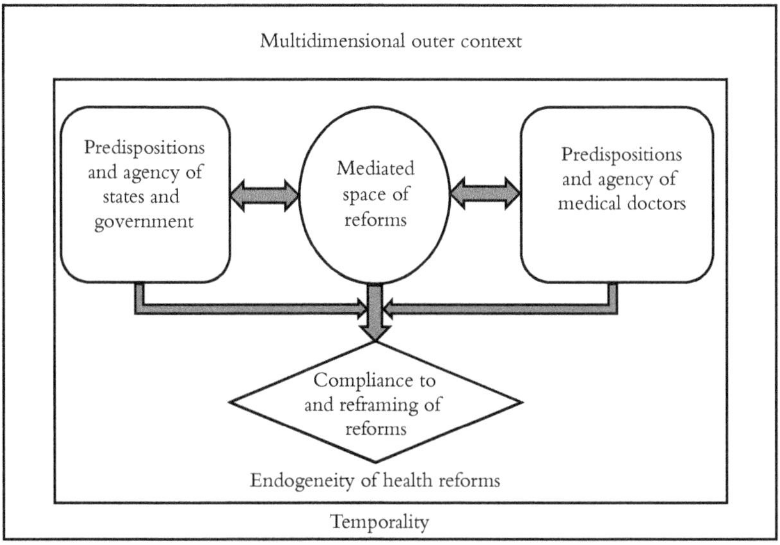

Theoretical model for comparative study of the role of medical doctors in healthcare reforms

Our conceptual model can be summarised as follows (see Figure 1.1). Context impacts in various ways on the development of reforms and the manifestation of agency in medical doctors and governments. Distal and proximal context variables influence the manifestation of agency of reformers and the medical profession. Proximal context interacts with and filters the influence of more distal contextual drivers. Proximal context refers to the endogeneity of healthcare systems conceived as an interactive and interdependent field generating its own dynamic, which shapes the content of reforms and the relations between various stakeholders. We propose that changes within healthcare systems promote greater alignment and interdependency between government and the medical profession. Consequently, medical doctors may simultaneously participate in the development of reforms and resist transformative policies. The hypothesis of growing interdependency between the medical profession and the State, along with political trends in mature welfare states, support a logic of co-production where medical doctors and governments embark in a common endeavour to meet emerging needs and system goals and face symmetric frustrations. Healthcare reforms are debated, framed and reframed within a negotiated space where a complex set of policies and instruments are proposed by government and eventually countered by medical doctors. The interaction between government and medical doctors within the negotiating space is associated with different policy instruments, including legal and economic instruments, in line with a more collaborative and co-productive approach to policy-making. Reforms open up a negotiated space in which government and the medical profession engage to shape and reshape narratives of change. Manifestations of the medical profession's agency within that space take various forms, from overt resistance and opposition to collaboration and co-production.

A key focus in policy exchanges and debates is around the 'what' – that is, the objectives of reforms (what problems need to be fixed) – and the 'how' – that is, the instruments or solutions selected. The becoming of reforms is largely influenced by active negotiation and mediation around these two aspects of reform. The manifestation of the collective agency of medical doctors is conditioned by the perceived impact on latent and manifest controls embedded in reformative templates. Power resources of both protagonists intervene in shaping relations and expressions of agency within the negotiated space. Co-production takes form within a complex pattern of relations between government and the medical profession. It implies that reforms are based on balanced considerations of the mutual concerns of governments and professions.

The resulting *real reform*, that is, the one shaped by the interactions and dual agency of government and the medical profession within the negotiated space, combines narratives of steering and narratives of dialogue in an attempt to balance government imperatives and the aspirations and expectations of the medical profession. This balancing act varies according to the salience of forces that inhabit the distal and proximal context and how key stakeholders interpret these factors and their urgency. According to our model, involvement and agency of medical doctors and governments within reforms is analogous to the performance of institutional work, and aims to maintain, transform or create new institutional templates that will shape the expression of medical professionalism within healthcare systems. Institutional work is fundamental to medical politics and aims to preserve professional ideals of autonomy and self-regulation in the context of insistent pressure for change. In this model, healthcare reforms are in a constant state of becoming, inhabited by drivers of change and stasis within the distal and proximal context and the interactive dynamics between two main interdependent actors: government and the medical profession.

Notes
[1]   https://scc-csc.lexum.com/scc-csc/scc-csc/en/item/1643/index.do
[2]   www.justice.gc.ca/eng/csj-sjc/rfc-dlc/ccrf-ccdl/

Research methodology: tracking the role of medical doctors in healthcare reforms

The objective of empirically exploring the role of medical doctors in healthcare reforms and policy changes raises a number of methodological questions. What data set should be considered? What is the appropriate period of study (that is, when should analysis of reforms start and end our)? What context-specific elements, whether jurisdictional or situational, influence agency in healthcare reforms? What characterises the roles played by various actors in the reform process? With what influence on context and policy outcomes? What methods should be used to compare case studies? These questions led us to consider methodological developments in *contextualist* and *process* research (Mintzberg and Waters, 1982; Pettigrew, 1987, 2012; Langley, 1999), which appear as a plausible way to approach policy research. We thus look at policy changes, such as healthcare reforms, as a continuing system in becoming (Pettigrew, 1987; Tsoukas and Chia, 2002). We rely on comparative longitudinal case studies (Fitzgerald and Dopson, 2009) to track the evolving dynamics of healthcare reforms and medical politics in two national empirical contexts: the NHS in England and the healthcare systems of two Canadian provinces: Quebec and Ontario.

Selection of the case studies in England and Canada

A number of logical arguments support the selection of these two national jurisdictions for our research. Both have a tax-based PFHS. Both have been fertile ground for healthcare reforms and are frequently selected as case studies in comparative health policy analysis (Tuohy, 1999, 2018). While England's PFHS predates those in Canada, they each span some 50 years, providing ample material for the study of healthcare reforms. They are both considered mature healthcare states (Tuohy, 2012) with free access to healthcare at the point of use, universal access and coverage, and the right to equality of treatment. Both jurisdictions also have a well-paid and well-trained medical profession, and medical doctors are considered key players and privileged interlocutors in reforms (Klein, 1990; Lazar et al, 2013). The healthcare systems in these two jurisdictions are highly regulated and centrally governed, even though medical doctors remain largely self-regulated. In both jurisdictions (although not exclusively so in England), medical doctors negotiate their participation in the system through organised and recognised bodies such as unions and professional associations.

Canada is a federation where legislative competencies are shared between two levels of government – federal and provincial or territorial (see Chapter 3). The regulation of healthcare systems falls mainly under the responsibility of the provinces and territories, although the federal level can use certain constitutional powers (notably its 'spending power') to influence provincial healthcare systems. To study healthcare reforms in Canada, we focus on the healthcare systems of the two largest sub-national jurisdictions (provinces) that together represent 61 per cent of the total Canadian population: Ontario (14.59 million) and Québec (8.48 million). Both provinces must – if they are to avoid financial penalties – adhere to federal health policies (notably the Canada Health Act) in the governance of their own healthcare systems. Yet these two provinces are seen over time to adopt various approaches to healthcare reform and policy change with potentially different impacts on the evolution and manifestation of medical politics. This provides fertile ground for comparative analysis.

Among the four countries of the United Kingdom, only England has all of its matters governed by central British institutions, and its National Health Service (NHS) is subject to the laws of the Westminster Parliament. Up until the 1999 devolution of power that provided the three other countries of the UK (Northern Ireland, Wales and Scotland) authority to organise and control their respective healthcare systems, laws governing healthcare applied to all countries in the UK. In England, the British government maintains the power to set top-level priorities for healthcare, and its Department of Health and Social Care provides NHS England with resources to plan and purchase services to assure universal access to the entire English population. At its foundation in 1948, the NHS was the world's first universal healthcare system financed with public funding.

Data sources

Empirical analysis of each of the case studies is based on primary and secondary data.

We first undertook a literature review of secondary sources, including academic journal articles, monographs and book chapters. We then reviewed the grey literature, including documents from government archives and professional publications from medical organisations.

With regard to primary sources, our research in England covers the period from the1940s until 2019. We found abundant scholarly work on healthcare reforms that integrated media accounts, and this was used to support our analysis. For the Canadian cases, an original analysis of media sources was needed starting from 1960, which also provided accounts of earlier sources going back to the 1940s. A systematic search of print and broadcast media was conducted to enrich the analysis of key policy debates and understand the power dynamics between the medical profession and government during reformative periods. In addition to the analysis of exchanges around proposed reforms, we relied on media reports or exchanges published five days before and five days after key policy events to document the medical politics at play in Québec and Ontario. For England, we conducted a general search using a snowball strategy from media sources cited in the literature, relying primarily on articles and commentaries published in the *British Medical Journal* (*BMJ*) as the main voice of the medical profession.

We also analysed policy documents that initiated reform processes, such as White Papers, Commission reports in Canada, and transcripts of parliamentary debates in both countries. These sources offered first-hand accounts of the medical profession's reaction to government policy proposals. position papers issued by professional medical bodies that detailed their response to proposed reforms were also included in the analysis.

A systematic search of legal documents relevant to each reform period was conducted. Bills introduced in Parliament, enacted laws, court rulings, contracts and collective bargaining agreements were studied to refine our analysis of the formalisation of each reform. We paid particular attention to the negotiation of Bills and the final version of adopted Acts, as these illustrate how legal instruments are mobilised during reformative periods.

Data analysis

Our approach to the analysis of empirical material involved the following steps:

1. Develop a theoretical model as a preliminary guide for empirical analysis (see Chapter 1).
2. Select and define core constructs of the theoretical model and generate a set of related concepts as heuristic devices to support the coding and interpretation of data (see the Appendix for definitions of key constructs, related concepts and strategies for empirical assessment).
3. Produce a preliminary chronology for each case to test our ability to reveal and assess the role of medical doctors in healthcare reforms. Two investigators coded key events and situations using the list of core constructs and related concepts and cross-validated findings through deliberation.
4. Write extensive descriptive individual case narratives (first-order analysis). Two investigators undertook this task, with systematic feedback from other members of the research team. Each narrative provides a timeline of reforms or major policy changes, with phases that constitute the unit of analysis, to empirically probe the role of medical doctors and

governments in the unfolding of reforms. Each phase is structured around (a) key events at various levels of analysis that form the distal and proximal context; (b) government proposals of healthcare reforms or policy changes; and (c) the responses and strategies developed by medical doctors and governments as reforms unfold.

5. Generate an analytical narrative for each case (*second-order analysis*) using a pattern–matching approach to assess the roles of medical doctors and governments in healthcare reforms. The analysis is iterative, with alternating phases of writing and interpretive sessions. Structured exchanges among members of the research team were used to validate interpretations and insights. Second–order analysis developed around three analytical dimensions: drivers and shapers of medical politics; strategies used by the two protagonists within the mediated space and their reactions to evolving situations and context; and consequential implications for medical politics and healthcare reforms.

   Steps 4 and 5 developed over numerous cycles to incrementally reduce the length of narratives while refining interpretations and insights.

6. Undertake comparative analysis of the three cases by confronting *second-order narratives*. In pairs, members of the research team performed the following analytical tasks: (a) identify convergence and divergence between the initial theoretical model and the within-case analysis; (b) calibrate the roles and weights of various drivers of healthcare reforms, such as contextual factors and strategies used by the two protagonists; (c) assess how interactions within the mediating space influence the trajectory of healthcare reforms and medical politics; and (d) summarise key lessons for the articulation and co-existence of healthcare reforms and medical politics in contemporary healthcare systems. Deliberations within the research team helped bring core insights to a higher level of abstraction and, ultimately, a higher level of theoretical generalisability. This analytical step culminated in a set of insights around the theoretical and research contributions of our work, and the policy implications presented in the book's Discussion and Conclusion.

Methodological reasoning and analytical logics

Our empirical inquiry focuses on the role of medical doctors in shaping health policies – taking the case of health reforms as a revelatory context for this phenomenon. As previously stated, the positions medical doctors adopt in relation to reformative propositions are based on a complex set of interests and values. In promoting a specific concept of reforms or priority for reforms, medical doctors share with governments and other stakeholders their interests and values, and reveal what it is they aim to achieve or defend in the context of a reform. While there are debates and uncertainties in sociology around the characterisation of and relationship between concepts of interests and values (Swedberg, 2005; Martin and Lembo, 2020), we consider that interests and values are driving forces that shape the strategies developed and positions taken by organised medicine and governments within the mediated space of reforms. In this research, we do not attempt to make a clear distinction between different types of interests and values. We empirically document manifestations of professional interests and values via an analysis of the discourse and position papers that medical unions, professional bodies and associations share in important arenas such as parliamentary commissions and debates and the press, including public campaigns and advertising. In promoting their views and defending their positions, medical doctors express their understanding of professional values and interests, including employment terms and working conditions. A similar approach is used to document the interests and values governments seek to promote or defend within reforms.

Our analysis also builds on an historical point of reference: the initial representation of the interests and values of medical doctors and governments during the creation of PFHS. We then track these over time to understand how interactions between these two groups evolve and shape their respective positions. In doing so, we recognise that interests and values – or at least their public manifestations during reforms – are not static, but rather, complex evolving patterns that respond to changes in the distal and proximal context, as described in our conceptual framework. Public declarations of what needs to be promoted or defended are considered powerful drivers of interactions and strategies during reforms.

Our analytical approach aligns with recent studies of contemporary medical politics and health policies. For example, Tuohy (2018), in her book on health reforms, highlights the importance of studying the agency of key actors or groups within relatively transient moments of opportunity for major change, such as reforms. In addition, she considers that in this type of analysis, one needs to rely on the disclosed preferences of actors or groups in order to understand strategic positions and assumptions that guide their involvement in policy-making. For Quadagno (2010), the development of welfare states provides fertile ground for the creation of groups dedicated to influencing policy agendas, including reforms. Quadagno explains that organisations representing medicine or medical doctors, such as professional bodies and unions, tend to apply major force in attempts to shape policy. Laugesen (2017), in her study of medical politics in the US around the payment of medical doctors, finds that the dynamic between governments and these organised entities is crucial to understanding the evolution of contemporary health politics and policies. Therefore, the focus of our inquiry is not on the views or behaviours of individual medical doctors, or on initiatives taken by sub-segments of the medical profession within their day-to-day practices.

Rather, our focus is on the role of organised medicine within the context of reforms, offering an admittedly partial but potentially impactful rendering of the views and roles of medical doctors in health policies and systems.

In summary, our research is structured around how medical doctors have strategically positioned themselves within the mediated space of reforms, and have influenced (or failed to influence) policy changes and/or side-lined core elements of reformative templates. By providing a detailed analysis of the interactions and exchanges between government and medical doctors, we unveil important aspects of policy changes. The agency and power of our two protagonists influences what makes its way into reforms and what is set aside. Our empirical objective is strictly focused on the interactions between two key actors in health reforms: the medical profession and government. We do not aim to analyse in a comprehensive manner the outcome of health reforms. Our analysis focuses on reforms as context and pretext for the expression of agency by medical doctors and the State. We intentionally exclude detailed analysis of the roles of other professions or groups such as the nursing profession and health managers in shaping health reforms. This methodological decision does not imply that other groups or professions lack significant influence in health reforms. In our analysis, we take into account the roles of these other groups when they are involved in debates and exchanges between governments and the medical profession about health reforms. We also pay attention to challenges arising outside the government-medical profession duality that influence policy formation. As will be seen in the empirical findings, we do not observe in our empirical cases that groups or professions apart from government have systematically challenged the position of the medical profession in health reforms (Alford, 1975). Where relevant, we have incorporated in our case narratives situations in which sub-groups of the medical profession have challenged the majority positions of their unions or professional associations.

The role of medical doctors in healthcare reforms in two Canadian provinces

The federal context

The federal context in Canada warrants attention as it influences the negotiating space for provincial governments and medical doctors. While healthcare services are mostly under provincial jurisdiction (Section 92, Constitution Act 1867), the federal government plays an important role, particularly by using its spending power to uphold national standards (for example, with respect to insurance coverage for services provided in hospital or by medical doctors via the Canada Health Act, 1985).[1] To various degrees and at different times in the history of Medicare in Canada, provincial governments have seen federal spending intervention as an attempt to exert control in a provincial domain (see Commission d'enquête sur la santé et le bien-être social, 1967–1972, for example). Frustrations were especially high when the federal government significantly reduced its financial contribution to provincial health systems during the recession of the 1990s (CPHA, 1995; Snoddon, 1998; BCMA, 2000: 14) while still requiring that provinces meet the same national standards.

Spending power is the federal government's main means of influencing provincial or territorial health insurance plans. As part of the reformative social policy agenda that emerged after the Second World War, the federal government adopted the Hospital Insurance and Diagnostic Services Act in 1957. Under the Act, the federal government would cover approximately 50 per cent of provincial and territorial expenses for hospital and diagnostic services, conditional on provinces or territories respecting criteria such as universality (such criteria would later be integrated into the Canada Health Act). As Medicare historian Malcolm Taylor describes, 'the majority of provincial governments, previously relatively unconcerned with the economic and health problems of their citizens, now had to face both an aroused public opinion and, for the first time, the prospects of the compelling pressures of provincial grants inducing them to action in an area clearly of provincial constitutional jurisdiction' (Taylor, 2009: 68). In 1966, the federal government passed the Medical Care Act. Again, the federal government would finance approximately 50 per cent of the costs of medical services provided in provincial programmes that met certain criteria. Ultimately, these federal Acts forced the establishment of publicly funded provincial health insurance regimes across the country between 1968 and 1972, primarily focused on curative care.

The federal Canada Health Act (CHA) deserves a few words here as a key piece of legislation in healthcare governance (with considerable influence on possibilities for healthcare reforms). In the early 1980s, the practice of user fees and extra billing, where medical doctors charge patients a fee over and above their Medicare payment, led to public frustrations and triggered considerable debate within the federal government (in Québec the practice was already illegal). The federal government proposed deducting extra billing and user fee amounts from federal funding under a new CHA to be introduced in the fall of 1983 (Ward, 1983). Federal Health Minister Monique Bégin met with provincial health ministers in September 1983, but despite strong opposition (notably from British Columbia [BC], Alberta and Ontario) they offered no viable counterproposal to the federal government's plan to discourage extra billing. The House of Commons in Ottawa gave the Canada Health Act, RSC, 1985, c. C-6[2] unanimous support (including from federal Conservatives). The CHA replaced the Medical Care Insurance Act and empowered the federal government to withhold a dollar in transfers to a province or territory for every dollar charged through extra billing and user fees (Sections 18, 19 and 20). The financing scheme between federal and provincial governments had evolved since the 1970s into a complex fiscal arrangement that combined determined sums of money (cash payments) based on GDP and population growth with a transfer of tax points (Tuohy, 1999).

In addition to formally prohibiting extra billing and user fees, the CHA specifies five criteria provinces or territories must meet in order to receive federal funding: (1) public administration of the health insurance plan (Section 8); (2) comprehensive coverage of all medically necessary hospital and medical services (Sections 9 and 2); (3) universal coverage (no group or person should be excluded) (Section 10); (4) 'portability', so Canadians remain covered even if they travel outside their home province or out of the country (Section 11); and lastly, (5) accessible care without direct or indirect barriers, including financial barriers.

The CHA has been at the heart of federal involvement in healthcare for nearly 40 years and has important symbolic value to Canadians (Romanow Commission Report, 2002). However, the fact that it has never been updated has triggered criticism, notably around its negative impact on the capacity of provincial healthcare systems to experiment with new delivery models and move away from overly hospital- and doctor-centred approaches (Régis

2008; Flood and Thomas, 2016). These parameters provide the federal context for healthcare reforms at provincial level.

Part 1: Québec case narrative

The 'prehistory': healthcare prior to the creation of Medicare, 1940–71

Prior to the creation of public health insurance programmes for hospitals and medical services that culminated in the single-payer Medicare system in Québec in 1971, healthcare services were mostly assured by private concerns, such as insurance companies, religious communities, and so on (Bélanger, 1992). Medical doctors practised their profession independently, maintaining control over payment and practice conditions (Desrosiers, 1986). The main oversight body was the College of Physicians of Québec (Collège des médecins du Québec, CMQ), which also represented the interests of the medical profession. The decades that preceded Medicare saw a shift from traditional individual practice arrangements towards a more organised form of medicine where the profession collectively pursued common objectives. This change was mostly due to increased specialisation in medicine and to the emergence and spread of unionisation in the medical profession (Dussault, 1975; Demers, 2003; Facal, 2006).

Specialisation appeared to destabilise the *modus operandi* of a profession that was until then relatively homogenous, at least in principle. The medical profession split into two distinct unions, respectively created in 1963 and 1965: the union of general practitioners (GPs), named the Fédération des médecins omnipraticiens du Québec (Association of General Practitioners of Quebec, FMOQ), and the union of specialists, named the Fédération des médecins spécialistes du Québec (Association of Medical Specialists of Quebec, FMSQ). In 1966, a third union was created for medical residents in Québec's medical schools, the Fédération des médecins résidents du Québec (Association of Medical Residents of Quebec, FMRQ). The Québec government formally recognised the role of the FMOQ and FMSQ in 1966 (*Agreement Relative to Medical Assistance* and Section 6 of the Medical Assistance Act), and they remain the only two interlocutors allowed to negotiate and conclude agreements with government on behalf of medical doctors (*Québec (Procureure générale) c. Guérin*, 2017, CSC 42; Section 19 of the Loi sur l'assurance-maladie). Following the creation of these two associations, the mandate of the CMQ was limited to overseeing and assuring the quality of medical practice.

Getting organised: pillars of the Québec Medicare structure

The Medicare system was created and implemented largely under the Liberal governments of Jean Lesage (1960–66) and Robert Bourassa (1970–76) during the 'Quiet Revolution'. This period was marked by the secularisation of government, reducing the influence of the Church, the emergence of the welfare state, and a general vibrancy in political, social and cultural life (Bélanger, 1992; Bourque and Leruste, 2010). Québec embarked on an ambitious programme to modernise its institutions, including in healthcare (Renaud, 1981; Guindon, 1998).

In 1966, the (conservative) Union nationale party was elected under Daniel Johnson. He quickly created the Commission of Inquiry on Health and Social Welfare, chaired by Claude Castonguay, to issue recommendations regarding whether Québec should fully join the federal plan to provide publicly funded medical services. In 1967, the Castonguay Commission issued a first report, which provided step-by-step recommendations for implementing a mandatory, universal, public and comprehensive healthcare insurance system. The report mentioned that the fee-for-service (FFS) payment method for medical doctors was not well aligned with the objectives of the new system (which integrated social or preventive and curative services) and instead suggested a salary model or payment based on the number of treated patients (Commission d'enquête sur la santé et le bien-être social, 1967–1972).

The CMQ expressed misgivings about the idea of a healthcare system based on 'free access' (Wuldart, 1966): the insufficient number of medical doctors would be problematic in a system that encouraged overconsumption of care. The CMQ demanded that additional medical faculties be created to increase the supply of medical doctors.

In 1969, under strong public pressure, the government created the Québec Health Insurance Board (Régie de l'assurance maladie du Québec or RAMQ – Québec Health Insurance Board Act, SQ, 1969, c. 53), as an arm's-length agency responsible for paying medical doctors. The two medical unions were not enthused about the creation of RAMQ as it had control over medical practice (Dutrisac, 1970a, b). To assure medical support, the government decided that RAMQ's board of directors would include representatives from the FMOQ and FMSQ. During parliamentary debates (it should be noted that in Québec the parliament is called the National Assembly), this representation was presented by government as an opportunity for medical doctors to have 'an oversight role' in the administration of the public insurance programme (Commission de la santé, Fascicule n°36, 1969).

In 1970, Castonguay became Minister of Social Affairs under the new Liberal government of Robert Bourassa. From this position, he led the 'Castonguay Reform' from 1970 to 1973, which laid the foundation for Québec Medicare. The main legislation, the Health Insurance Act (LQ, 1970, c. 37), stated that all costs related to services medically required by a resident of Québec and delivered by a medical doctor would be paid by RAMQ on an FFS basis (Sections 3 and 4). It also prohibited selling private insurance for 'insured services' covered under the public plan (Section 12). The goal was to avoid creating a parallel public/private regime and to encourage medical doctors to enrol in Medicare, as they would no longer be able to claim fees from private insurers. This legislative measure later proved to be quite effective in keeping medical doctors affiliated to the public system and set the scene for intense bilateral exchanges between government and medical doctors across various periods of reform. Any medical doctor could withdraw from the public payment scheme (Section 20), but the law gave the Minister of Health the power to force medical doctors to participate in the public system if the number of participating doctors was deemed insufficient (Section 24).

Before and after the adoption of the Health Insurance Act (which was modified in October 1970), medical associations were very vocal in expressing their concerns (and sometimes their support) about Medicare and discussing the conditions for their involvement. The FMOQ specified conditions under which they would agree to participate in the public regime: their position would not be inferior to specialists, FFS remuneration would apply to all medical doctors, they would have access to positions in academic health centres, and they would receive the same remuneration as specialists for a same medical act (Dussault, 1975; Facal, 2006; Savard, 2017). Expressing the collaborative mood at the time, FMOQ President Dr Gérard Hamel stated: 'We agree with the principles of the current bill, just as we agreed with the principles of the previous bill. Whether the law itself is good or not, the Fédération des médecins omnipraticiens du Québec remains willing to negotiate, because we are eager to collaborate to bring in a system that will remove the financial barriers that, in too many cases, stand between sick people and doctors' (National Assembly Debates, 1970a; our translation). The government eventually agreed to many of the GPs' requests.

In contrast, the FMSQ expressed strong opposition to the creation of the publicly funded system, considering that it would threaten professional autonomy. It was especially opposed to any form of forced participation (or limits to non-participation) in the system. During parliamentary debates, FMSQ President Dr Raymond Robillard said:

> the ability to withdraw from the regime is for us a crucial, essential, necessary thing. ... About the right to withdraw, we consider that there is a need to preserve the doctor's freedom. We want doctors to join the plan and we have organised ourselves – and we are the only ones in Canada to do so – in a union to negotiate with the government, something doctors in other provinces have refused to do, in order to join the plan. We want to join a plan voluntarily. (National Assembly Debates, 1970a; our translation)

The specialists considered that the conditions of the insurance programme 'imposed by authority, therefore arbitrarily ... affect the fundamental conditions of the practice of medicine and impact doctors' right to negotiate their working conditions' (Dutrisac, 1970a: 4; our translation).

Government and the public grew irritated by the specialists' objections. They were perceived as 'the spoiled children of the future insurance plan' who were 'manipulating the government' (Roy, 1970: 2; Ryan, 1970: 3; our translation). The Prime Minister declared that 'the government will not give in to blackmail' and 'with the hundreds of millions of dollars we've invested in the hospital sector, the doctors should be the last to resort to blackmail to force the government to change a plan that it considers in line with public interest' (Dupre, 1970: 1, 8; our translation). Castonguay suggested appointing a mediator, which proved unsuccessful as the FMSQ and government could not even agree on the scope of the mediator's mandate (National Assembly Debates, 1970b). Specialists called a strike that began on 7 October 1970. Along with the right to withdraw, a major issue in the specialists' strike was the ban on extra billing included in the Act (Tuohy, 1999).

The strike coincided with a major political and social crisis, the 'October Crisis' (La crise d'octobre), when the Front de libération du Québec (FLQ), a radical sovereignist political organisation, kidnapped a British diplomat and a government minister. The two events, the FLQ and the creation of Québec Medicare, became historically linked. The government, preoccupied by the political crisis, sought better collaboration from the specialists (Facal, 2006). With other actors already prepared, under various conditions, to participate in the public plan, the specialists' continued opposition left them isolated and the government adopted the final measures of the Medicare regime without their approval. The Act to Amend the Health Insurance Act (SQ, 1970, c. 38), adopted in October 1970, completed the Medicare reform in Québec. Medical doctors could choose from among three types of status (which still exist today): 'participant' status for medical doctors fully participating in the public system (Section 1[b]); 'withdrawn professional' (or 'disengaged') status for medical doctors who practice outside the public system but agree to charge patients the same fees as the public regime (Section 1[b²]); and 'non-participant' status for medical doctors who work outside the public regime and set their own fees (Section 1[b³]. The government also forced an end to the strike by imposing heavy fines and penalties through the adoption of a special law for specialists (Act respecting medical services 1970). In November 1970, the FMOQ reached an agreement with the government concerning professional fees under the public regime (*La Presse*, 1970, A1, A6). The FMSQ reached an agreement on fees in January 1971.

During the Medicare reform, the government clearly gave up on the salary model proposed by the Castonguay Commission. A few years later, Castonguay (no longer Health Minister) said during a conference that he had made that choice because he was managing resistance on different fronts and could not cope with turning medical doctors against him as well considering the political power they could mobilise (Bélanger, 1992). Following this reform, the government committed to forego reliance on legislation or regulation in managing medical doctors' remuneration, and instead proceeded through negotiated bilateral agreements with the FMSQ and FMOQ. This commitment held for many years, until it was disturbed by the Barrette reform of 2014.

The implementation game, 1971–80

The early 1970s were characterised by a series of consultations and bills (including projet de loi (PL) 65, Loi de l'organisation des services de santé et des services sociaux) to give concrete form to the new publicly funded health system. Minister Castonguay wanted to design structures and rules that would formally delineate the roles of the medical profession within publicly funded healthcare organisations (for example, the role of GPs in emergency departments). He also proposed creating a Regional Organisation of Social Affairs (Organisation régionale des affaires sociales, or ORAS) with regulatory powers to inspect and investigate medical practice.

Aspects of the Bill that challenged the existing roles and autonomy of medical doctors were highly criticised by the medical profession. The CMQ opposed ORAS and fought to preserve self-regulation by the medical profession and its own role in quality assurance and inspection (Richard, 1971). Specialists reacted strongly to the possibility of losing control over the organisation, distribution and control of their practices and to the bureaucratisation of healthcare (FMSQ-LS, 2015a: 25). They expressed a fundamental credo that no reform would be possible without their collaboration (FMSQ-LS, 2015a: 25). The FMOQ voiced its opposition in similar terms and sought genuine involvement in shaping the new system (Chalvin, 1971; Daoust, 1971; Commission permanente des affaires sociales, Bill 65, 5 October 1971). During parliamentary debates, the FMOQ's President, Dr Hamel said:

> We believe that physicians must have the right, at some point, to express their perception of needs … that they are perhaps best able to determine, discern these needs, assess them, etc. And that relates, of course, to our recommendation that physicians participate at all levels where decisions are made. … Our desire to be present on boards of directors must be seen as a desire to participate, as a desire for dialogue. (Our translation)

In December 1971, the Act respecting health services and social services proposed the creation of a council of medical doctors, dentists and pharmacists (CMDP) in each hospital that would report directly to the board of directors on matters related to the quality of professional practice and care. Castonguay argued that this council, which was mostly composed of medical doctors, was not an administrative body, but would control quality of care. This proposal was well received by the FMSQ as it addressed medical doctors' concerns regarding their role and autonomy (FMSQ-LS, 2015a: 25).

Furthermore, after two years of negotiations, the FMSQ obtained a new contract with government that alleviated concerns regarding the evolution of specialist remuneration (FMSQ-LS, 2015a: 26). However, the FMSQ had to accept the idea of a global ceiling on medical compensation (Fournier and Contandriopoulos, 1997), showing the ability of the government of the time to impose some of its policy objectives in relation to medical doctors.

Strain and conflict, 1980–90

Public finances were a major source of concern for the Parti Québécois government in the 1980s. The salaries and social benefits of civil servants were reduced. Growing healthcare costs and reduced federal transfers raised questions about the sustainability of the healthcare system (Bélanger, 1992). This period was associated with efforts to rationalise the system and with increasing attempts by government to impose new bureaucratic controls on medical services.

During 1981–82, the government and medical unions were engaged in intense cycles of negotiations to define the working conditions of medical doctors and residents. Unions developed pressure tactics such as work slow-downs, boycotting administrative and teaching activities and general strikes. For GPs and specialists, the issue was not just compensation, but also the imposition of bureaucratic control on medical practice (including quotas on their workload and obligations to practice in remote areas). Specialists and GPs were aware that their compensation compared unfavourably to other provinces. After a general strike by GPs in 1982, the government imposed a 14 per cent increase in compensation (GPs were asking for 47.4 per cent) (Gingras, 1982: A3; des Rivières, 1982: A3). The FMSQ negotiated a parallel agreement with government (Roberge, 1982b). While the FMRQ was mobilised at various points during these negotiations, residents considered their demands were only partially heard (Roberge, 1982a). They participated with GPs in the general strike. While this period of conflict dealt mostly with medical compensation, the problem of sufficient distribution of medical services across the province persisted. The government launched a Commission under Jean Rochon to look at the functioning and financing of the healthcare system.[3]

In 1985, the Liberal Party was elected with a majority government. In 1988, the Rochon Commission released its final report, which proposed shifting from a healthcare system 'held hostage by providers' to a system focused on population health. The report explored societal transformations and healthcare system dynamics that could achieve a major realignment around the objective of health and wellbeing at population level. This broad perspective implied that no specific group or organisation, including the medical profession, should dictate health policies and the rules that govern the day-to-day functioning of the system. While the Commission's perspective was novel, the report was deliberately vague on specific solutions to implement the vision: 'With this report, the Commission aims to provide all persons and interest groups in the field of health and social services with a new basis for discussion, exchange and debate. It thus hopes to provide an opportunity to establish a new balance in power relations that might refocus the system on its real objectives' (Rochon, 1988: xii; our translation). The report did not garner much reaction from the medical profession, perhaps because it did not raise any controversial issues regarding medical compensation. The medical profession was virtually absent from public media following the report's publication.

The 1980s saw another period of tension between the medical profession and government. A strike by medical residents to protest their working conditions (some trainees were working for 24 to 36 hours at a stretch) culminated in an order from the Essential Services Council (Conseil des services essentiels) that forced them to return to work (Noel, 1987). In November 1987, the FMRQ and government signed an agreement that included the creation of a bilateral committee to assess the working conditions of residents and propose improvements (Beaulieu, 1987).

Finally, in spring 1988, the new Minister of Health and Social Services, Thérèse Lavoie-Roux, organised a cross-province consultation based on the Rochon Commission report to identify tangible ways to operationalise its vision. Following the consultation, she detailed a proposal for healthcare system reform in a White Paper entitled 'Pour améliorer la santé et le bien-être au Québec: Orientations' Ministère de la Santé et des Services sociaux [MSSS], 1989). It presented a diagnosis of the healthcare system and suggested approaches to various challenges and issues. Regarding medical services, the document insisted on the need for strong regulation around the distribution of medical doctors, between GPs and specialists and across the territory, to ensure fair access to healthcare services.

Tensions and flirtations in medical policy, 1990–2000

Bill 120 (Act to amend the Act respecting health services and social services and other legislative provisions) was introduced in 1991 to reform the healthcare system. Key elements of the Bill were presented in a White Paper entitled 'Une réforme axée sur le citoyen' ('A citizen-centred reform').

Among other elements, it clearly promoted integrating the medical profession more closely into the system (MSSS, 1990: 12). During the parliamentary commission to discuss the Bill, Minister Marc-Yvan Côté (1989–94) stressed the need to achieve a better balance between the needs of the population and the autonomy of the medical profession regarding the location of practice: 'For my part, I am keen to ensure that Québeckers in the regions receive medical services because they pay the same taxes as people in Montréal, Québec City or elsewhere. The bill does not call into question the fundamental freedoms of doctors, contrary to what has been conveyed. We believe that it strikes a fair balance between individual freedoms and collective responsibilities' (National Assembly Debates, 1991; our translation). Côté went on to present a long and detailed description of the many amendments made to the Bill in order to respond to objections from the medical profession, insisting on government's good will. The FMSQ expressed opposition to the Bill's mandating specialists to practice in underserved areas (FMSQ, 1991), asking instead for an incentive-based and non-coercive system to solve the problem.

In the summer of 1991, medical unions formed a coalition to oppose Bill 120. They launched a campaign in which they portrayed the healthcare system being captured by bureaucrats. A series of pressure tactics, such as 'study days', were used. Medical doctors advocated for a reform like Ontario's, where a joint government–medical profession committee was created to provide advice on the delivery of care. Minister Côté announced that the reform would be adopted despite the profession's objections. The response from the medical profession was bold, with media campaigns comparing bureaucrats, calm and aloof, to medical doctors on the ward lacking the materials they needed to save lives (Paré, 1991). Medical unions eventually met with the Prime Minister and obtained assurance they would be consulted on all aspects of Bill 120 in exchange for stopping their pressures tactics. This period culminated with the removal from the Bill of any provisions related to the distribution of medical services across the territory and the inclusion of a guarantee that medical doctors would participate on the boards of hospitals and healthcare organisations. The agreement between medical unions and the government was eventually signed, enabled by intervention from the Prime Minister. Overall, 439 amendments were made on the 494 sections of the Bill (Giroux et al, 1999). The reform also created the Regional Medical Commission (Commission médicale régionale) and the Medical Council of Quebéc (Conseil médical du Québec), an advisory body composed mostly of medical doctors with a mandate to make recommendations to government on the organisation of medical services.

Increasing healthcare costs and issues around access to care triggered another round of reforms in 1996. Following the election of a Parti Québécois government in 1994, Dr Jean Rochon (of the Commission) became Minister of Health and Social Services (1994–98). A major healthcare reform was launched to respond to cuts in federal health transfers, to support a shift to ambulatory care, and to fulfil a political ambition to achieve a zero deficit in order to prepare for the political independence of Québec. This reform reduced hospital capacity through hospital mergers and closures, encouraged early retirement of an important contingent of healthcare professionals, including medical doctors, and imposed severe budget cuts (Fournier, 2001; Denis et al, 2006).

The reform was very difficult for healthcare managers and staff, but did not directly target the medical profession, except that they had to deal with the pressures on staff and services associated with austerity policies and the redistribution of medical workforce. Resistance was less evident among GPs than specialists – the FMSQ declined an invitation from government to participate in the parliamentary commission (FMSQ, 1996), and associations representing the younger segment of the medical profession (FMRQ, 1996: 2, PL 116). The FMOQ was collaborative (FMOQ, 1996: 1, PL 116), although they stressed that medical doctors in private clinics played a crucial role in the delivery of care and should receive proper consideration in any reform. They were also adamant about maintaining the participation of medical doctors in the governance (public boards) of publicly funded healthcare organisations (FMOQ, 1996: 7, PL, 116) The reform (Bill 116, Act to amend the Act respecting health services and social services) was finally adopted in June 1996 without too many amendments, revealing the government's determination to reorganise the system. The medical profession voiced its concerns, but was not able to temper the government's reformative ambition. A significant number of medical doctors retired from practice following this reform.

Other reform ideas were promoted through Bill 404 (Act to amend the Act respecting health services and social services and amending various legislative provisions) adopted in 1998, to complete the 'Rochon reform'. The FMOQ again reacted quite positively to the proposed reform. It saw the Bill's creation of regional directorates of GPs (Direction régionale de médecine générale [DRMG]) – a structure within the regional health authority (RHA) led by a GP and dedicated to the planning and organisation of general practice – as an opportunity to increase their role in health policy (FMOQ, 1998: 35, PL 404). The FMSQ strongly opposed what it saw as excessive bureaucratic control in the system (FMSQ, 1998: 1–2, PL 404) and advocated for a much more significant role in governance and decision-making processes that impacted on medical practice and services. They considered that government was not receptive to this idea, and sought to make the general population more aware of their views (FMSQ, 1998: 3, PL 404). They emphasised the unique role of health professionals, specifically the medical profession, and the natural rights they have in the healthcare system considering they are the ones treating disease and patients (FMSQ, 1998: 4, PL 404).

A different and somewhat discordant note in medical politics was struck by a new professional association created in 1995, the Québec Association of Young Doctors (Association des jeunes médecins du Québec, AJMQ). They criticised the conservatism of the medical college and unions and were preoccupied with maintaining the social and moral engagement of medical doctors and with the importance of fighting as a profession for the integrity of the publicly funded healthcare system (AJMQ, 1998: 6, PL 404). They also objected to excessive control by bureaucrats of the system, and considered coercive measures to force young medical doctors to practice in underserved areas as inappropriate. The association launched a class action suit in 1997 to oppose an agreement signed between the government and the FMSQ that forced young specialists to practice in the regions (AJMQ, 1998: 6–7, PL 404).

Negotiations with various medical groups culminated in Bill 404 being adopted with amendments that mostly aligned with the views of medical unions and associations. The medical profession became more integrated into the governance and management structures of healthcare organisations and RHAs (the DRMG), while maintaining their autonomy and assuming new roles in advising government (the Direction des affaires médicales du MSSS, formed in 1999). Minister of Health and Social Services, Pauline Marois (1998–2001), stated in 1999 that these new bodies would restore the participation of medical doctors in major decisions regarding the healthcare system.

Collaboration and confrontation, 2000–13

In 2001, the Clair Commission report was released with proposals for healthcare reform. The Commission received its mandate from the leadership of the Parti Québécois (1996–2003), a government recognised for its socially progressive policies.

The Position Paper presented to the Commission by the FMSQ mentioned concerns with access to care, and suggested that while the publicly funded system should be maintained, a larger role might be given to private clinics or private financing (FMSQ, 2000a: 3). The FMSQ proposed creating a dedicated fund for the healthcare system, considering that government administration of the regime was inefficient (FMSQ, 2000a: 4, 93), and advocated increased investment in healthcare to address past rationalisation (FMSQ, 2000b: 6). They also, in a letter to the Canadian Prime Minister, asked that the federal government restore its financial participation in provincial healthcare systems to pre-cutback levels (FMSQ, 2000a: 7). The FMSQ was supportive of reforms to reinforce the role of primary care doctors and introduce more coordinated and integrated approaches to care (FMSQ, 2000a: 9, 10). Finally, they demanded greater involvement in and control over the management of the healthcare system (FMSQ, 2000b: 14), including the implementation of a permanent bilateral committee for manpower planning in medical specialties (Lettre d'entente no 129, Annexe 11, between the Minister of Health and Social Services and the FMSQ, April 2001).

By supporting a reinforced role for GPs and integrated primary healthcare organisations, the FMSQ was in line with reforms that would be enacted in 2003 by a newly elected Liberal government (2003–12), and Health and Social Services Minister, Dr Philippe Couillard (2003–08). Yet the FMSQ resisted any intervention that would force specialists to practice in underserved areas (FMSQ, 2000b).

The Clair Commission report aimed to identify concrete solutions to current dysfunctions in the Québec healthcare system. The Commission recommended the creation of primary care groups called Family Medicine Groups (FMGs), in which a core group of GPs, along with nursing staff and administrative support, would develop more effective models of care delivery. The Commission also recommended the creation of affiliated specialist clinics that would sign contracts with publicly funded healthcare organisations. The report specified that medical doctors' compensation should promote the development of these clinics (Clair report, 2000: 55, 86). It also stressed the need to better value the roles of the medical doctors in the system and involve them more in decision-making around the organisation of care (Clair report, 2000: 101): Overall, the Clair Commission report was well received by the medical profession.

Following the Clair Commission report, the Parti Québécois' Minister of Health and Social Services, Rémi Trudel (2001–02), introduced Bill 28 (Act to amend the Act respecting health services and social services and other legislative provisions), which aimed to strengthen the role of RHAs in the governance of the healthcare system and the integration of medical doctors in the governance of healthcare organisations. The FMOQ expressed satisfaction with the government's intention to guarantee medical doctors a presence on the boards of publicly funded healthcare organisations (FMOQ, 2001: 3, PL 28). The FMSQ reasserted the crucial role of specialists in the development of healthcare policies and the importance of joint mechanisms to govern the system, including medical services (FMSQ, 2001: 1, 3, PL 28). The FMRQ saw Bill 28 as coherent with the Clair Commission report, and stressed the importance of having nurses and medical doctors represented on boards and of reinforcing board accountability (FMRQ, 2001, PL 28). Bill 28 was rapidly adopted.

In 2002, a crisis arose as hospitals, and hospital emergency departments especially were short of staff, with 11 hospitals in the province at risk of being unable to maintain services. The crisis introduced a very tense period in relations between the government and the medical profession. The Minister of Health and Social Services, François Legault (2002–03, Parti Québécois), was determined to fix the problem, even if this meant forcing medical doctors to provide services in at-risk hospitals. The Minister threatened medical doctors with a special law (Bill 114, Act to ensure the continued provision of emergency medical services) to oblige medical doctors (mostly GPs) to work in underserved areas and keep hospital emergency departments open across the territory. The three medical unions (FMOQ, FMSQ and FMRQ) joined forces to oppose the special law (FMOQ, FMSQ and FMRQ, 2002), and mentioned that problems of access would not be resolved with coercive measures; solutions required joint policy-making efforts. Medical unions met with the Prime Minister to try and prevent the law, but it was nevertheless adopted in a divided National Assembly on 25 July 2002.

In August, medical unions informed the government that they would contest the special law in court (Sirois, 2002b). The FMSQ undertook a series of pressure tactics (study days, disengagement from teaching and administrative activities, work slow-downs) to arrive at an agreement with the government around their labour contract. Their pressure tactics led to 10,000 medical procedures being delayed (Sirois and Breton, 2002). FMSQ opposition was followed by intense negotiations to find a viable solution for hospitals unable to guarantee access to emergency services. Meanwhile, the FMOQ signed an Agreement with government that improved GPs' practice conditions in emergency departments. In February 2003, the FMSQ and the government agreed that Bill 114 would not apply to specialists. The Agreement provided specialists with a significant increase in remuneration along with funds to support additional volumes of specialist medical procedures. In the 2014 settling of a class action suit organised by a group of patients (Conseil pour la protection des malades, CMP), the Québec Court of Appeal obliged the FMSQ to pay CAN$837,750 plus interest to compensate patients who suffered delays in access to care due to pressure tactics used during the 2002 conflict (*Fédération des médecins spécialistes du Québec vs Conseil pour la protection des malades*, 2014, QCCA 459).

In November 2003, the newly elected Liberal government announced the so-called 'Couillard reforms'. These were driven by three main objectives: (1) limiting the growth of health expenditure in the context of an ageing population; (2) improving the coordination and continuity of care to better respond to the needs of vulnerable populations; and (3) placing more emphasis on preventive health in addition to treating illness (Cloutier et al, 2006).

The government presented Bill 25 (Act respecting local health services and social services network development agencies) in the hope of significantly restructuring the healthcare system. The FMOQ agreed with the objectives of the reform (FMOQ, Position Paper on Bill 25, December 2003). Bill 25 focused on the voluntary creation of territory-based local health networks under the leadership of organisations formed through the merger of small hospitals, long-term care centres, and local community health centres. Medical doctors in private clinics were invited to join these networks. However, they doubted the system's ability to use family medicine appropriately and saw private clinics and FMGs run by GPs as an opportunity to invest and engage in the integration of care (FMOQ, 2003: 7, PL 25).

The FMSQ clearly stated their disappointment with a reform based on structural changes. In contrast to the FMOQ, they recognised the importance of consolidating structures, but worried about a reform that was more administrative than clinical. They also insisted on the principle that medical doctors should guide any reorganisation of care (FMSQ, 2003: 6, 11, PL 25). Ultimately, the FMSQ's position was more in line with the Clair Commission recommendations than with Couillard's reform.

Overall, the 2003 reform and measures that followed it were relatively well received by the medical profession. However, they remained concerned with difficulties ensuring sufficient resources in the healthcare system. In 2005, the Supreme Court of Canada ruled in *Chaoulli vs Québec* ((Attorney General) [2005] 1 SCR 791) that government had to be effective (including in respecting people's right to life and security) in managing the healthcare system and assuring timely access if it was to lawfully restrict access to private healthcare. The ruling prompted a segment of the medical profession to create Québec Doctors for a Public System (Médecins Québécois pour le regime public, MQRP), a political movement to protect publicly funded healthcare in Québec.

Bill 83 (Act to amend the Act respecting health services and social services and other legislative provisions), introduced in 2004 and adopted a year later, was an opportunity to work on various aspects of the reform and enable policy exchanges between government and the medical profession. The FMOQ considered that the Bill limited patient choice and freedom to select their medical doctor, and also constrained the freedom for medical doctors to accept patients (FMOQ, 2005, PL 83). However, they appreciated the government's decision to rely on GPs and their private clinics to achieve better integration of care and services in the system (FMOQ, 2005, PL 83: 15). The FMOQ emphasised that medical doctors should be well represented and active in RHAs to inform the organisation of care. They resisted attempts to develop regulations for the quality of medical practice that went beyond those of the CMQ (FMOQ, 2005, PL 83: 18).

The CMQ presented a pessimistic view of the reform, saying that it did not uphold the promises included in Bill 25. They saw the reform as centralisation and bureaucratisation, and not as moving towards a system centred on patient needs. They detected a government determination to 'discipline' healthcare organisations and providers (CMQ, 2005: 2, PL 83), and did not see the value of adding regulatory and inspection mechanisms to those already applied by the CMQ.

In 2006, the government published a White Paper, *Guarantee of Access to Care in the Québec Healthcare System* (MSSS, 2006: 60), which responded, in principle, to the *Chaoulli* case. This opened up options for private medical clinics to partner with public healthcare organisations. Both medical unions supported this orientation, while also applauding the government for maintaining strong support for the publicly funded system (FMOQ, 2006, PL 33; FMSQ, 2006). Adopted in December 2006, Bill 33 created the legislative conditions to formally recognise the role of private clinics in the provision of publicly funded care.

In 2008, Dr Yves Bolduc became Minister of Health and Social Services under the Liberal government. His term was characterised by an attempt to optimise the delivery of care, relying on the Lean management approach. While a distinctly managerial turn, the idea of optimising efficiency through LEAN did not seem to raise significant opposition from medical unions.

Doctors in the driver's seat, 2014–18

The Barrette reform included a series of Bills (Bill 10, 20 and 130) that aimed to improve access to care and services as well as increase efficiency in the healthcare system. Access was an important source of dissatisfaction among Québeckers, who faced long wait lists for elective treatments, long waits in emergency departments, and difficult access to medical doctors outside hospitals.[4] The reform started in 2014, following the election of the Liberal Party with Dr Couillard as Prime Minister and Dr Gaétan Barrette as Minister of Health and Social Services (2014–18). A specialist himself (radiologist), Barrette was President of the FMSQ before the election. This unprecedented situation led to much speculation about how he would deal with the healthcare system and medical doctors.

Barrette presented the first part of the reform as dedicated to 'facilitate and simplify public access to services, improve the quality and safety of health care and make the network more efficient and effective' (Explanatory Notes, Bill 10, 2014). The proposition was to reduce the number of bureaucrats in the system and give the Minister 'new powers with regard to regional and supraregional institutions, in particular the power to prescribe rules relating to their organisational structure and management' (Explanatory Notes, Bill 10, 2014). Barrette considered that reducing the size of the system's governance infrastructure would help achieve his objectives. RHAs (regional level) would be eliminated, leaving two levels: the healthcare institution (local) and the Ministry (central). Furthermore, the number of healthcare institutions would be significantly reduced by assembling various facilities under common institutional governance.

Before details of the Bill were made public, medical groups welcomed the general idea behind Barrette's reform. The new President of the FMSQ, Dr

Diane Francoeur, stated 'it is music to our ears' as they had been asking for years to shed bureaucratic weight (Daoust-Boivert, 2014a).

However, medical doctors changed their position when Bill 10 (Act to modify the organisation and governance of the health and social services network, in particular by abolishing regional agencies) was made public, details of the reform were unveiled and the parliamentary consultation process began. Medical unions immediately complained that the one-month limit to comment the Bill was too short (see, for example, FMSQ, 2014: 3, PL 10, FMOQ, 2014: 5 , PL 10) and that the Bill concentrated too much governance power in the hands of the Minister. The FMSQ pointed out that the reform gave the Minister a 'blank cheque' and 'unprecedented power' to manage the system as he saw fit. The Minister would be able to nominate all members of the board of directors in healthcare institutions, effectively increasing the politicisation of the healthcare system (FMSQ, 2014: 11, PL 10; Ouellet, 2014). Regarding the government's increased regulatory powers, including the power to intervene directly in the management and structure of healthcare institutions, the FMSQ stated: 'We are witnessing quasi absolute government power over regulation. This is unprecedented!' (FMSQ, 2014: 11, PL 10; our translation). The MQRP denounced Minister Barrette's 'autocratic tendencies' and the CMQ described the reform as 'a 19-wagon train with a single engine, the ministry, and a single conductor, the minister' (Daoust-Boisvert, 2014b; our translation). The FMOQ, while applauding the abolition of RHAs, was concerned by the creation of oversized healthcare institutions that could have a negative impact on medical resources management and responsiveness to patient needs (FMOQ, 2014: 4, 6, 8, 9, 12 , PL 10). Other medical groups shared this concern about supersized institutions (ACMDPQ, 2014: 6; CMQ, 2014: 6, 9; FMSQ, 2014: 5, PL 10). The FMOQ was also disappointed that GP contributions were not recognised in 'institutional affairs' as they could not be appointed to the board of directors of the new institutions – the CISSS and CIUSSS. 'It's maddening to see the government deny the presence and contribution of thousands of GPs in running these institution' (FMOQ, 2014: 10, PL 10; our translation). The FMOQ described the reform as akin to placing the entire province under guardianship (Daoust-Boivert, 2014b).

Following the parliamentary consultation process, the government changed some aspects of the Bill, while maintaining key objectives. Modifications were made to the composition of institutions' boards of directors, enabling GPs to become members, and a specific seat on the board was reserved for a specialist (Section 9). The Minister also agreed to be less intrusive in appointing board members. However, the Minister preserved the additional regulatory powers, along with the power to temporarily replace a CEO (Section 152) and control 'medical workforce plans' (Section 91).

The second phase of the Barrette reform, Bill 20 (Act to enact the Act to promote access to family medicine and specialised medicine and to amend various legislative provisions relating to assisted procreation) was introduced in November 2014. The government sought to optimise medical and financial resources and improve access to family medicine and specialised medicine (Explanatory Notes, Bill 20). The government's main strategy to achieve this objective involved increasing the productivity of medical doctors and improving timely access to medical services. The Bill imposed new individual duties on medical doctors that, if not fulfilled, would lead to financial penalties (up to 30 per cent of their income). GPs would have to provide medical care to a minimum caseload of patients and perform a minimum number of hours of medical activities. The Bill required specialists to 'provide medical consultations, elsewhere than in the emergency department of an institution, to a minimum number of patients' (Section 10) and to provide services 'to users that have been registered under the specialist's name for over six months on the access list' (Section 12). This Bill provoked major criticism from all medical associations. It gave the Minister the power to change the conditions of remuneration on an individual basis. This represented a major disruption of the negotiated approach to medical doctors' remuneration that had been in place since the inception of Medicare.

In 2015, Bill 20 was debated in parliamentary sessions and medical associations were highly vocal during that process, including in the public sphere. The CMA wrote:

> This is the first time that the CMA has submitted a brief to the National Assembly of Québec, and it is also the first time that the QMA (Québec Medical Association) and the CMA have submitted a joint brief. This collaboration speaks volumes about the concerns physicians across the country have about Bill 20. This bill constitutes an attack on the professional autonomy of physicians unprecedented in the history of organized medicine in Canada. There is no doubt that it concerns the entire medical profession as this bill could have major consequences for the medical profession. (AMQ and CMA, 2015: 3; our translation)

The FMOQ launched a media campaign with headlines such as 'Bill 20 is the cancer of general medical practice' (*La Presse*, 2015a, A6, 2015b, A5, 2015c, A6) and a message to government: 'The Federation calls on the government to renounce the abuse of power. We demand that Bill 20 be withdrawn and invite government to sit down with us to negotiate change and choose to implement constructive solutions' (FMOQ, 2015a: 4, PL 20; our translation). At least three medical faculties declared a strike at the end of March 2015 to oppose Bill 20 (Lacoursier, 2015: A8).

The FMSQ strongly opposed the Bill, ultimately demanding its total withdrawal. It further expressed doubts as to the government's intention to take their opinion into account during the consultation process (Nadeau, 2015a). The FMSQ referred to the Bill as a 'coercive approach that infringes on medical doctors' rights', an 'abusive use of regulatory powers' and a 'contemptuous approach' to medical doctors which also denies them their right to negotiate (FMSQ, 2005a, PL 20; Nadeau, 2015b). When the FMSQ presented its position in oral hearings at the Commission, discussions with the Minister were acrimonious on both sides (National Assembly Debates, 2015a).

The FMOQ eventually opted for a more collaborative approach and invited the Minister to discuss with GPs how to ensure better access to medical services. Among various propositions, the FMOQ suggested the creation of 'superclinics' to unclog emergency departments in hospitals (Nadeau, 2015b, c; National Assembly Debates, 2015b) and develop interprofessional collaborative practices. The FMOQ also made a commitment on behalf of its members to take on more patients, as requested by the Minister. As FMOQ President, Dr Godin stated, better to do this than to manage the 'mess' Bill 20 will create (Nadeau, 2015b, c).

On 25 May 2015, an agreement in principle was reached between the FMOQ and the Ministry confirming that Bill 20 would not apply to GPs (Agreement in principle concluded between the FMOQ and the Ministry to increase and improve the accessibility of primary care medical services). This further involved GPs in the management of medical resources as well as the definition of 'particular medical activities' and medical workforce plans. The FMOQ committed its membership to assuring that 85 per cent of Québeckers would have a family doctor by 31 December 2017. The Bill was not withdrawn, as the agreement brought just a suspension of its application. Despite this agreement, bitterness about Bill 20 lingered among GPs. In November 2015, Dr Godin said:

> in the political debates surrounding this bill worthy of the Soviet era, we have heard many slanderous statements tinged with unfounded prejudices against family physicians. The outcome of the new law is already extremely negative: uncertainty in the medical world, devaluation of family medicine, a counterproductive climate of confrontation of between the State and doctors and the State's attempt to dehumanize primary care. (FMOQ, 2015a; our translation)

Similarly, on 11 January 2016, an agreement in principle was concluded between the FMSQ and the Ministry confirming the non-application of Bill 20, with a few exceptions regarding the management of the medical workforce (Agreement in principle between the FMSQ and the Ministry to increase and improve the accessibility of specialist medical services). The FMSQ took on the commitment to achieve the Ministry's accessibility targets.

Bill 130 (Act to amend certain provisions regarding the clinical organisation and management of health and social service institutions), introduced on 9 December 2016, and adopted on 26 October 2017, is the third major piece of the Barrette reform. Following on Bill 10, it aimed to amend certain rules around boards of directors and the assistant president and executive directors (APED). It specified that APED would be appointed by the government, on the recommendation by the Minister of a candidate selected from a list of names provided by the institutions' board of directors. The Bill also changed certain rules relating to medical governance in healthcare institutions, notably regarding the appointment and privileges of medical doctors who practice in such institutions. The Bill stipulated that the Minister could impose an access system for specialised services that every public healthcare institution would have to follow. In addition, various internal rules in healthcare institutions would have to be authorised by the Minister, including rules coming from the CMDP, which had the role of assessing and assuring the quality and pertinence of medical acts performed in the institution. Finally, the Bill allowed the Minister to impose a central access system to specialised medical services, put in place by RAMQ.

During parliamentary consultations on Bill 130, medical associations criticised various aspects of the Bill. The Québec Medical Association (Association médicale du Québec, AMQ) asked that more power be given to medical doctor managers based on the principle of medical professionalism and clinical governance, rather than weakening the medical–management partnership (AMQ, 2017: 4). This position was echoed by the CMQ, FMOQ and FMSQ (CMQ, 2017: 2, PL 130; FMOQ, 2017: 14, PL 130, FMSQ, 2017: 22, PL 130).

The most contested points of the Bill were, first, that the Minister could require boards of directors to impose additional duties on GPs and specialists in order for their institutional privileges (allowing them to practise in the institution) to be renewed. Second, the Minister could influence regulation of the internal organisation of healthcare institutions, such as the board of directors or the CMDP. This was viewed as an additional loss of professional autonomy (Richer, 2016). Barrette agreed that this represented a loss, yet claimed it was for the benefit of patients (Chouinard, 2016). The President of the FMSQ pointed out that the Minister had once again chosen to impose unilateral legislative measures instead of working with specialists, which painted the profession in a negative light (*La Presse*, 10 December 2016[5]). The FMSQ highlighted the frustrating pattern of the Barrette reform:

As with Bills 10, 20, 92 and 118, the minister is using this bill to give himself a host of new powers, as if the powers already conferred on him by current laws were not sufficient to enable him to adequately perform his duties. Passage of this bill will add to the minister's powers of intervention, which are already excessive, if not abusive. In addition to posing a real danger of misuse, the concentration of power in the hands of one person opens the door to an extreme politicization of the healthcare system. This tendency, entrenched as the National Assembly adopts these many pieces of legislation, goes against recognised rules for the sound governance of public institutions. (FMSQ, 2017: 3, PL 130; our translation)

The FMSQ initiated legal proceedings to oppose certain decisions they considered illegal based on unauthorised use of power by the Minister (Marin, 2017). As for the FMOQ, while supported in its desire to partner in policies aiming to improve efficiency and access to healthcare services, the reform introduced an exaggerated need for control by a Minister who sought to subject medical doctors to his will (Chouinard, 2016; FMOQ, 2017: 4–5, PL 130).

As with Bill 20, agreements in principle were concluded with both medical unions regarding the non-application ('moratorium') of certain sections of Bill 130. The government agreed not to regulate management of the medical workforce in healthcare institutions or add obligations for medical doctors to obtain or renew their privileges. The FMSQ was the first union to conclude an agreement. It accepted to withdraw legal action (Entente MSSS–FMSQ, Section F(i)) and to work with the Health Ministry to put together a joint committee to formulate recommendations on various topics related to the organisation of care and the conditions of medical practice (Entente MSSS–FMSQ: 2–3). In May 2018, the FMOQ issued a press release mentioning it had concluded an agreement with the Ministry. It also agreed to create a joint committee with the Ministry to explore and make recommendations on rules relating to the management of the medical workforce and GP roles and conditions of practice in healthcare institutions (Entente de principe sur la Loi 130, press release, 18 May 2018).

Part 2: Québec case analysis

The 'prehistory': healthcare prior to the creation of Medicare, 1940–71

The influence of context: drivers and shapers of medical politics

Following federal healthcare policy initiatives, Québec's government explicitly set out to establish a comprehensive publicly funded health service, launching the Castonguay Commission (Commission d'enquête sur la santé et le bien-être social, 1967–1972). The socioeconomic context during that period created favourable conditions for the newly elected Liberal government (1960–66) to embark on an ambitious programme to modernise the State and Québec society with the development and legitimation of secular institutions (Bélanger, 1992; Bourque and Leruste, 2010). This period, which extended into the 1970s, was influenced by the 'Quiet Revolution' and benefited from broader economic, technological and scientific developments. The increasingly specialised knowledge and technical sophistication of medicine required more industrial forms of healthcare organisation (Dussault, 1975), demanding greater financial and human resources. This endogenous evolution of medicine heralded a new era in which the State's emerging welfare agenda converged with the development of modern medicine. The evolution of the medical profession toward greater specialisation also created a context that favoured political differentiation within the profession, between GPs and specialists.

Strategies used by the protagonists to deal with the evolving context

During the 1960s, the medical profession took its first steps to organise itself to deal with a government that was more active and interventionist in the healthcare arena. The profession had mixed feelings about the prospect of a public healthcare system; while it would offer protection from bad debts, it would also create a permanent interdependence between the medical profession and the government. As they began to negotiate the conditions for participation in the emerging public system, medical doctors recognised they needed to develop a collective and representative voice (Facal, 2006). This led to the establishment of three medical unions: the FMOQ for GPs, the FMSQ for specialists and the FMRQ for medical residents. For government, this unionisation was an opportunity to limit interactions during the negotiating process to a few specific groups. The formal recognition of these unions delineated the negotiating space, occupied primarily by the FMOQ and FMSQ.

The government's main strategy for developing health policies was to set up a commission (the Castonguay Commission) to evaluate the current state of healthcare services and make policy recommendations regarding the implementation of a publicly funded system. The Commission provided a space where various stakeholders and experts could express their views and preferences on proposed changes that responded to the federal government's promotion of publicly funded healthcare. It placed the medical profession at the forefront of a strong political trend, fuelled by federal policies, toward publicly funded healthcare. The FMOQ, representing GPs, welcomed the creation of a publicly funded healthcare system, seeing it as an opportunity to enhance their status and working conditions (Dussault, 1975; Facal, 2006). They expressed their willingness to collaborate in the creation of a system that reduced barriers between patients and medical doctors (National

Assembly Debates, 1970a). The FMSQ, representing specialists, viewed the idea of such a system as an attack on professional autonomy and was reluctant to accept rules that would bar specialists from receiving payments through private insurance (Dutrisac, 1970a: 4). The government was astute in defending the principle that medical doctors had to choose between practising in the public regime 'in becoming' or opting out and relying on private payment without the intermediary of private insurance (which the government would make illegal for services covered by the public regime) (Health Insurance Act, SQ, 1970, c. 37). The population and the public press were not very sympathetic to the concerns of specialists, and support withered when the specialists' strike.

Overall, this period created a mediated space where two protagonists, the government and the medical profession, could play their political game. A fundamental structuration of medical politics also emerged, based on the differentiation of GPs from specialists, and a schism emerged between them in defending the interests of the profession. The medical profession organised to give itself a voice during reforms that affected the financing of medical care, yet specialists were not able to counter the strong political and public forces driving the installation of a publicly funded system. Medical politics was, in a way, formalised and sanctioned by government as part of this new public system. The government legally recognised the FMSQ and FMOQ as the sole official negotiators for the medical profession, and committed to managing medical doctors' remuneration through negotiated bilateral agreements rather than regulation. The medical profession emerged with the political tools (including political representation and formal negotiating power) to navigate this new health policy landscape.

Implications for medical politics and healthcare reforms

This period in health policy in Québec shaped the healthcare system and the medical political institutions that have persisted to this day. The government achieved its policy goals by putting in place a framework conducive to the design and implementation of a publicly funded healthcare system. The medical profession progressively became a quasi-public profession through its involvement in the development of the publicly funded system, despite formally remaining a private provider (unlike most healthcare professionals). In setting the parameters of the new healthcare system, the government granted the medical profession its preferred model of compensation – fee-for-service – and guaranteed medical doctors autonomy in setting up and managing their private clinics while being paid by public funds. This period also established that the provision of medical care in hospitals and clinics would form the core of the public system, with less place for a community approach to health. At the end of the day, a major reform creating Québec's public healthcare system came hand in hand with the fabrication of a medical politics that appeared more conservative than reformative.

The implementation game, 1971–80

The influence of context: drivers and shapers of medical politics

The 1970s saw the implementation of, and adjustments to, Québec's newly created publicly funded healthcare system. It was marked by endogenous dynamics that impacted the framing of medical doctors' concerns and government attempts to negotiate a *modus operandi* for the system. The growing cost of healthcare (now more accessible to Québeckers), including important increases in medical compensation, raised government concerns around the long-term viability of the system (Contandriopoulos et al, 1989). In addition, reductions in federal contributions for healthcare led to growing awareness among provinces that they would have to bear most of the responsibility for financing these new public systems. These endogenous and exogenous factors associated with the economic downturn (the oil crises) of the early 1970s encouraged the government of Québec to develop strategies that would ensure the proper integration and regulation of medical doctors' practice.

Strategies used by the protagonists to accommodate and deal with the evolving context

This period saw considerable debate around the design and implementation of the publicly funded healthcare system. While government aimed to introduce regulations over and above professional self-regulation, the medical profession saw this as excessive bureaucratic control and feared being absorbed into a system that had already significantly increased government power. The medical profession's response indicated they were open to joint governance of the system and felt that reform was not possible without their collaboration (FMSQa, 2015: 25; Chalvin, 1971; Daoust, 1971). In the end, the government retreated from most attempts to regulate medical doctors, while achieving some formalisation of control over medical practice within hospitals. In negotiating compensation, the government was able to implement a global ceiling mechanism to contain the overall cost of specialist compensation. Negotiations with the FMSQ were long and difficult but government was nevertheless able to assert its status as single payer of medical care and services (Fournier and Contandriopoulos, 1997).

Implications for medical politics and healthcare reforms

On the one hand, developments in the 1970s demonstrate the government's ability to pursue a reform project with the collaboration of medical doctors.

On the other hand, medical doctors came on board with many caveats and demands around preserving their special status and autonomy. The mediated space constructed in the 1960s became the stage on which the government and the medical profession played their political games (that were often quite confrontational). The tension between the challenges of operating a healthcare system and the aspirations of the medical profession to join government at the helm of the system became explicit as medical doctors gained a voice. Medical doctors mostly accepted the new rules of the game and integrated their practice within the publicly funded healthcare system. The system institutionalised the 'double bed politics', striking a deal at the outset that recognised the interdependence between government and medical doctors. However, segments of the medical profession, notably specialists, remained sceptical about 'bureaucratic rationalisers' and sought joint governance that valued medical doctors' specific expertise, power and perspective. Medical politics in Québec during this period is marked by the ambiguous position of medical doctors who were supportive, in practice, of the PFHS, but reluctant to rethink their role, status and practice within this new context.

Strain and conflict: learning to dance in step, 1980–90

The influence of context: drivers and shapers of medical politics

Political, economic and legal imperatives played a key role in framing the relationship between medical doctors and government in the 1980s. The economic recession and rising interest rates in Canada had a major impact on the financial situation of provincial and federal governments. At the federal level, this context and increasing healthcare expenditure led the government to lower the proportion of provincial healthcare expenses it would cover (Bélanger, 1992). The context of economic austerity did not, however, moderate the expectations of the medical profession. Endogenous forces also exerted pressure on the Québec health system. The experiences of the previous decade revealed how costly it was for government to provide universal access to healthcare in the face of scientific and technological progress. In addition, the architecture of the healthcare system – reinforced by the CHA that guaranteed universal access to 'medically necessary services provided by doctors or in hospitals' – strengthened the privileged and strategic position of medical doctors (Régis, 2008). As independent professionals (very rarely employees), paid by public funds, medical doctors' structural position reinforced their autonomy and power within the healthcare system. Representation by well-organised unions enabled them to capitalise on this unique position and heightened their bargaining power. Ultimately, interactions between the medical profession and government during this period revolved around competing expectations and imperatives, revealing underlying tensions between the government's responsibilities (including its fiscal responsibilities), and the autonomy and collective aspirations of medical doctors. This tension would recur in later periods. Aspirations were not always homogenous within the medical profession, with GPs and specialists often speaking with quite distinct voices.

Strategies used by the protagonists to accommodate and deal with the evolving context

The government tried to contain the cost of medical compensation through various strategies such as increased bureaucratic control or the rationalisation of medical practice. It relied mostly on coercive policy instruments: for instance, Bill 91 (1982) imposed working conditions on GPs and Bill 15 (1984) prohibited extra billing. The medical profession, through their unions, reacted strongly to the imposition of bureaucratic controls and quotas, and used various pressure tactics (including a general strike by GPs in 1982). Medical doctors were positioned to assert their views within the mediated space, but also instigated the political game with government by interacting directly with the public through media campaigns. Another strategy was to compare their remuneration with that of medical doctors in other provinces. Medical doctors saw themselves as part of a broader collective that could act outside the mediated space for negotiations between medical unions and government. With GPs, the government ended up using coercive means to impose working conditions and set remuneration (des Rivières, 1982: A3; Gingras, 1982: A3). Medical politics appeared especially fragmented during this period. The FMSQ decided to negotiate its own agreement, rejecting the idea of a political alliance with the FMOQ. The FMRQ voiced its views, but was a marginal player at the bottom of the medical profession's pecking order.

Tensions between the government and medical unions fuelled talk of establishing a commission, viewed as a collaborative policy tool, to take stock of the healthcare system and its evolving dynamics. A commission was seen by the Parti Québécois government as a way to step back from the heat of medical politics and broaden the conversation around the future of the system. It was an opportunity to move beyond the 'behind closed doors' conversations that were typical of the bilateral relationship between medical unions and government. The Rochon Commission report (1988) concluded that the healthcare system should be at the service of patients and, importantly, promote the health of the population and not just the development of medical services. The Commission expanded the political landscape behind the mediated space by integrating new voices and new considerations into conversations around healthcare reforms (Rochon, 1988: xii). The government, while recognising its interdependence with the medical profession, sought to transcend 'double bed politics' in order to recalibrate power within the mediated space.

The medical profession had little to say about the Rochon Commission report, but medical unions voiced recurring themes in medical politics during this period, notably their scepticism of bureaucrats' ability to adequately run the healthcare system. In 1987, medical residents represented by the FMRQ used their right to strike to highlight the risks of a hospital system that relied on excessive overtime by medical residents.

Liberal Minister Lavoie-Roulx pursued a further round of consultations in 1998 with various stakeholders and citizens to develop plausible policy options based on the Rochon Commission report. The Minister aimed to increase accountability in the system and government's ability to manage the system. Policy ideas at the time reveal a growing determination to integrate medical doctors into joint policy-making (an approach akin to govermentalisation of the State) with government, but this co-existed with determination to preserve the core role of medical unions as defenders of the interests and autonomy of medical doctors.

Implications for medical politics and healthcare reforms

This period revealed a fundamental pattern that would become an enduring feature of medical politics in Québec. The government attempted to make the system more manageable and accountable, which required integrating medical doctors and getting them to participate in health policy-making. The 1980s were less a period of reform than of becoming acquainted, where each protagonist voiced their expectations and tested their ability to attain their goals, learning and adjusting along the way. The mediated space became a revelatory context, displaying the strength of a developing institution – labelled as medical politics – within the ecosystem of a PFHS, where the confrontation of views was channelled (primarily, although not exclusively) into a formal and relatively confined space. In a fragmented medical polity where GPs and specialists played their own political games, the medical profession was able to voice discontent and concerns and appeal to the public in hopes of expanding their influence in policy-making and improving their status and working conditions. The government was portrayed as an illegitimate bureaucratic rationaliser interfering with a benevolent medical profession. It had clear intentions to initiate reforms using various policy instruments, but was not running the political show; this was reflected in the Rochon Commission's limited impact on medical politics. Changing the institutions of medical politics could not be achieved in one strike as the institutional mechanisms in place protected a specific representation of the status and autonomy of the medical profession.

It takes two to tango: tensions and flirtations in medical policy, 1990–2000

The influence of context: drivers and shapers of medical politics

The economic recession of 1990–91, coupled with high levels of federal debt in Canada, led to an austerity agenda that saw federal contributions for healthcare fall even more dramatically than in previous periods (Snoddon, 1998). In Québec, the government sought to provide a coherent and transformative response to the Rochon Commission in order to increase pluralism within the healthcare system and make the system more responsive to citizens' needs. Persistent problems assuring access to medical care in underserved areas became a source a frustration. The government was driven by a consumerist ideology, where the system was expected to be more reactive to population needs and assure equal access across regions (National Assembly Debates, 1991). These different factors motivated reforms and created the conditions for open tensions between the medical profession and government. In addition, the Parti Québécois government (1996–2001) decided that the sovereignty agenda would be better served by eliminating Québec's public deficit, which led to cutbacks in healthcare (Paré, 1996).

Strategies used by the protagonists to accommodate and deal with the evolving context

The 1990 White Paper (*'A citizen-centred reform'*) clearly stated the Minister's intention to gain traction on the functioning of the healthcare system. Despite government assertions that the current *modus operandi* of the healthcare system was unacceptable (March 1990: 64, 8, 9), medical unions successfully opposed aspects of the reform that would force them to practice in underserved areas. Tensions between professional autonomy and universal access became tangible. Medical doctors advocated for positive incentives and joint policy-making to solve these issues. The FMSQ's conservative agenda was revealed in nostalgic public statements about the support and respect they used to enjoy as specialists (FMSQ, 1991: 25–6). Despite political orientations that were not totally aligned (the FMOQ generally endorsed a more collaborative approach with government), medical unions came together in 1991 to firmly oppose the government's reform proposal. They used a variety of pressure tactics that highlighted the risk of medicine being controlled by bureaucrats, but also more collaborative strategies such as direct negotiations with the Prime Minister. The government's response was to pull back and remove from the proposed bills most of the controversial sections that had the potential to constrain medical doctors (Giroux et al, 1999). The government also agreed to allow formal representation of medical doctors on the boards of major healthcare organisations. In addition, the principle of joint policy-making between the government and the medical profession was institutionalised with the creation of Regional Medical Commissions and the Medical Council of Québec.

In a second wave of reforms during the 1990s, rationalising public finances was at the top of the policy agenda (Fournier, 2001; Denis et al, 2006). The medical profession seemed relatively immune to these changes. In restructuring, the government did not attempt to change the relationship between medical doctors, organisations and the healthcare system, or alter their working conditions directly. The FMOQ's only complaint was that the reform did not sufficiently recognise private clinics as a major source of care (FMOQ, 1996: 1, PL 116). The FMSQ was concerned that the reform provided government more control over the system and called for healthcare managers to have less control and more accountability.

Implications for medical politics and health reforms

In reforms of the mid-1990s, the government was able to impose restructuring and budget cutbacks without much resistance from the medical profession. Reforms earlier in the decade were more problematic: they attempted to reinterpret the principle of the autonomy of the medical profession in order to resolve issues around access to care. The medical profession strongly and successfully opposed this reform, while also achieving government commitment to collaborative policy-making on medical affairs. The 1990s clearly revealed the duality of medical politics, where one source of power and agency lay in the formal regime of labour relations based on the principle of a bilateral monopoly between the government and the medical unions. This regime was often confrontational. The other pillar of medical politics was the negotiation of specific mediating spaces for joint policy-making, where medical unions (and the FMSQ most insistently) sought input into the policy-making process. These spaces were usually collaborative and ensured that medical doctors shaped the policies and regulations that would apply to them. These confined mediated spaces produced varying results, including the acceptance by medical doctors of some government imperatives. Acceptance was conditional on medical doctors feeling they had a voice and agreed on the policy objectives. These joint policy committees or governance bodies such as DRMGs were in some case the outcome of fierce initial opposition by the medical profession to proposed policies or reforms. Yet they ultimately provided an alternative to confrontational medical politics.

Changing moods: collaboration and confrontation, 2000–13

The influence of context: drivers and shapers of medical politics

The end of the 1990s introduced a period of relative prosperity in Canada, with inflation and public debt under control at the federal level. While that meant more stability in healthcare contributions, the federal government also sought to make some funding conditional on achieving improvements in provincial healthcare systems (Marchildon, 2013). In 2001, a new Prime Minister (Bernard Landry, Parti Québécois) was elected in Québec and stated that changes were needed to address problems in the healthcare system. The Clair Commission was mandated to propose concrete options for reform, in a spirit of increasing the healthcare system's agility and responsiveness. There was a feeling that the healthcare system could be better managed, and primary care improved. This was a period of optimism about what could or should be done to improve the healthcare system. Yet, in 2002, optimism soured as a major crisis in assuring emergency services in hospitals raised the thorny issue of medical services distribution (Sirois, 2002a: A2; *La Presse*, 2002: A3). The government was determined to fix the problem, and ensure better distribution of the medical doctors across the province. In 2005, the government was also forced to react to the Supreme Court ruling in *Chaoulli vs Québec* ([2005] 1 SCR 791), which recognised that excessive waiting times in the public system infringed on fundamental rights.

Strategies used by the protagonists to accommodate and deal with the evolving context

The government relied on a public commission to explore avenues for reform, which eventually led to legal changes that increased medical doctors' participation in system governance (for example, on the boards of healthcare organisations). The FMSQ saw the Clair Commission as an opportunity to promote the value of a publicly funded healthcare system along with some deregulation to provide the system more breathing room (FMSQ, 2000a). Specialists supported enhancement to the role of family medicine and better primary care services. They advocated governance renewal to replace bureaucratic structures with structures that would add value to the coordination and delivery of care (FMSQ, 2000b). The FMOQ was very supportive of reforms proposed by the Clair Commission and saw a new appreciation for their role and profession in the idea of FMGs (FMSQ, 2001, PL 28). They also highlighted the medical profession's participation as an ally in finding solutions to system difficulties.

In response to the emergency department crisis of 2002, the government threatened the medical community with a law that would force them to cover underserved areas. The Minister added that he intended to work on another Bill that would change medical doctors' status: 'The current status of autonomous entrepreneur is problematic as it allows doctors to work when they want, where they want, without a real connection to the network' (*Le Devoir*, 2002: A8; our translation).

Medical unions joined forces and issued a press release to oppose the coercive measure (Vollant and Senikas, 2002: A1–2; Sirois, 2002b: A14). The FMSQ appealed to the principle of professional autonomy and mobilised members to undertake pressure tactics (Breton and Sirois, 2002: A1; Sirois, 2002c A4; Sirois, 2002d: A3). An 'Operation Major Concern' day was organised at the Olympic Stadium in Montréal, where some 3,000 specialists assembled to express their opposition (Sirois, 2002b: A6). In December 2002, the government adopted Bill 142, which provided both negative and positive incentives for medical doctors to provide service in underserved areas. After intense negotiations, the government and the FMSQ concluded an agreement in early 2003 that exempted specialists from the law and awarded them a significant increase in compensation. The FMOQ appeared more compliant or collaborative, and concluded an agreement before the specialists. Overall, while both unions were committed to preserving professional autonomy and resisted coercive measures, each union negotiated an agreement with government that matched their particular views and interests.

Medical doctors' reactions to the Couillard reforms in 2003–05 were in line with previous patterns. The FMOQ expressed reservations about some aspects of the reform, but were generally collaborative (FMOQ, 2003, PL 25). The FMSQ found the reform disappointing as it focused on structural changes that offered little clinical benefit (FMSQ, 2003, PL 25). All medical unions opposed limits on the freedom of patients and medical doctors. Despite these objections, the medical profession did not mount any concerted opposition to these reforms.

In 2006, in response to the *Chaoulli* decision, the government published a White Paper (*Guarantir l'accès: Un défi d'équité, d'efficience et de qualité* [*Assuring Access: An Equity, Efficiency and Quality Challenge*]) promoting greater participation of private clinics in the delivery of publicly funded care. The FMSQ was determined to play a more important role in managing the delivery of medical care and the contribution of private clinics. The FMOQ fully supported the idea of using private clinics and of allowing additional financing through private insurance to cover some types of care (FMOQ, 2006, PL 33; FMSQ, 2006). This position was coherent with the predominant organisational model of GP practices (private clinics), but somewhat surprising considering their commitment to retain a monopoly over primary care.

This period of relative harmony between the medical profession and the government was interrupted in 2006 when medical specialists engaged in another round of tough negotiations around compensation. The government turned to the Essential Services Council to legally oblige specialists to fulfil at least some of their obligations, such as training medical residents. Both parties agreed to mediation to resolve the conflict, which culminated in further increases in specialist compensation.

Implications for medical politics and health reforms

The story of the 2000s repeated many elements seen in earlier reform periods. When reforms or policy shifts did not directly impact the medical profession and doctors' working conditions, the government was able to drive significant changes in the system. The corollary was that, for any reforms that touched on the medical profession and medical practice, the government had to negotiate and reach compromises with the medical profession. In terms of medical politics, the FMSQ appeared highly organised to voice the specialist position and resist reforms or policies they deemed unacceptable. In this period, the medical profession sought a much greater role in the system through their private clinics. While this was an opportunity to bring them on board and have them play a more active role in reforms, it also presented considerable risks for the government in terms of political acceptability.

Devils and heroes: doctors in the driver's seat, 2014–18

The influence of context: drivers and shapers of medical politics

This period was marked by recovery from the financial crisis in 2008 and a sense that the province's economic situation had improved. With the election of a new Liberal government in 2014, a period of major reforms began with the nomination of Dr Barrette, a medical specialist and past president of the FMSQ, as Minister of Health and Social Services. Dr Barrette appeared as a real political beast: he had strong views on the healthcare system and was eager to fight with all categories of personnel, including medical doctors, to accomplish his reforms. Minister Barrette considered that the healthcare system suffered from too many bureaucrats, a view that shaped his desire to merge publicly funded healthcare organisations and his proposals for improving access to care and efficiency in the healthcare system.

Strategies used by the protagonists to accommodate and deal with the evolving context

Minister Barrette proposed ambitious reforms, starting with Bill 10, which aimed to reduce the number of managers in the healthcare system while creating larger structures for them to manage. While medical unions were not happy with the short timeline for commenting the Bill (arguably part of the Minister' strategy) and the increased power the Minister gave himself in the reform, they applauded the move to reduce bureaucracy. The Minister was able to introduce the Bill without significant interference from medical doctors. During this period, the government's strategy involved a rapid and assertive pace of change, followed by negotiations when pressure reached the boiling point.

Minister Barrette then set out to increase the productivity of the medical profession, setting specific targets and financial penalties in Bill 20. Medical doctors became much less enthusiastic. They perceived that these measures posed a threat to their autonomy, implied a lack of trust in their ability to solve problems in the system, and further centralised power over healthcare in the government's hands. They vehemently opposed the reform and the Minister's 'authoritarian' leadership style, which was incongruent with the negotiation model (FMSQ, 2015b; *La Presse*, 2015a, b, c). The mediated space was tumultuous during this period, with intense exchanges, frequent use of regulatory powers, as well as heated negotiations between government and medical doctors. The Minister recognised the status and relevance of the medical profession as the core of a healthcare system, but was determined to gain more control, and exact greater efficiency and accountability from medical services.

The high visibility and fighting spirit of the Minister created a unique atmosphere around relations between government and the medical profession. Yet, the objectives pursued by government and the reactions of the medical profession were very much in continuity with previous reforms. Medical unions demanded collaborative or joint policy-making instead of coercion. They also blamed the government for problems in the healthcare system. In the end, both medical unions reluctantly concluded agreements with the government. The FMOQ managed to preserve self-regulation in exchange for a promise to meet productivity targets within an agreed timeline (Agreements on principles 2015 and 2016).

Minister Barrette's third major reform (Bill 130) sought to regulate the management of the medical workforce in healthcare organisations. This was perceived as a major affront as it collided with deeply held principles: professional autonomy and the medical profession's unique ability to solve healthcare system problems. The positions of the FMOQ and FMSQ on Bill 130 appeared to be closely aligned (FMOQ, 2017, PL 130; FMSQ, 2017, PL 130). Negotiations culminated with the government agreeing not to implement many of the new measures, but also led to the creation of joint policy committees involving the two main medical unions and government. The mandate of these committees was to explore and formulate recommendations on the organisation of care and the conditions of medical practice.

Implications for medical politics and healthcare reforms

This period illustrated the importance of distinguishing manifestations of agency from the impact of actions. A politically astute and courageous Minister with intimate knowledge of medical politics could not, on his own, significantly impact the status and role of medical doctors. Medical doctors were destabilised when faced with the Minister's determination to change the way doctors related to the system, but this did not dampen their determination to fight for important principles. The resulting reform was somewhat binary: the government (1) achieved major changes in the healthcare system outside the playing field of medical doctors and (2) managed to effect modest tangible changes in the medical profession's relation to the system. This situation once again highlighted a fundamental element of medical politics: medical doctors must buy into reforms at some point in the institutionalised bargaining arena. Demands for joint policy-making went hand in hand with positive (and not coercive) incentives. While 'double bed politics' were well entrenched, sleeping with the enemy was still an attractive option when, from the point of view of the medical profession, there was so much to gain.

Part 3: Ontario case narrative

The inception of Ontario Medicare: reconciling expectations, 1956–69

The political landscape in Ontario at the inception of Medicare was somewhat monochromatic, notably because the Progressive Conservative Party of Canada's (PC) reign in the province extended from 1943 to 1985. The Department of Health was headed by Dr Matthew Dymond (1958–69) during the early implementation of the PFHS. The creation of Ontario Medicare was strongly influenced by federal legislative initiatives; yet, unlike most other provinces, Ontario was initially intent on creating an alternative plan that would strike a compromise between the federal government's objectives and the interests of private insurers and organised medicine.

Following the federal government's adoption of the Hospital Insurance and Diagnostic Services Act, the Ontario government formed the Hospital Services Commission in order to assess the pertinence of creating a public hospital insurance programme. The Ontario Hospital Insurance Plan, introduced in 1959, did not cover services rendered by medical doctors. At that time, insurance for medical services was mostly provided by Physicians' Services Incorporated, a medical doctor-sponsored insurance company created and administered by the Ontario Medical Association (OMA), which represented both GPs and specialists.

In 1963, the OMA Council voted to 'initiate discussions with the Government of Ontario, with a view to implement an enlarged Medical Welfare Plan' (Holloran, 1990: 59). In 1965, with the support of the medical profession, the province adopted the Medical Services Insurance Act (Bill 136, 1965, c. 70), which concretised that idea of Medicare for all 'without regard to age, physical or mental infirmity, financial means, or occupation'. The Act also created the Medical Services Insurance Council (MSIC), in which two out of nine representatives would be nominated by the OMA (section 3(1)). At the Federal-Provincial Conference in July 1965, Ontario Premier Robarts was told by the federal government that the plan described in Bill 136 would not meet federal criteria of universality and portability and would therefore not be eligible for federal subsidies (*Toronto Star*, 1966b). The Ontario government then explored ways to modify Bill 136 to meet federal requirements and proposed the Act to amend the Medical Services Insurance Act 1965 (Bill 6, 1966/SO, 1966, c. 86).

In January 1966, the OMA sent members a declaration contesting numerous aspects of the new government plan and received 4,500 signatures (*Toronto Star*, 1966a). The declaration sought reaffirmation of the right for medical doctors not to participate in the plan, demanded a fee schedule 'developed by a responsible and autonomous profession, (that) is not open to negotiation nor proration with anybody or group', and insisted that 'neither the OMA nor an individual physician should enter, under any circumstances, into a contractual agreement with government in the area of medical services insurance' (*Toronto Star*, 1966a). Minister Dymond responded: 'I'm ashamed that the profession would use this method', and pointed to the cooperative stance of doctors in BC (*Toronto Star*, 1966a).

Finally, the Act to amend the Medical Services Insurance Act became law in February 1966. The amended Act created the Ontario Medical Services Insurance Plan (OMSIP), a government insurance agency responsible for overseeing its application. This was 'a blow to the OMA's ability to regulate the medical care needs of the people of Ontario' (Holloran, 1990: 88).

The OMA resisted some aspects of the provincial programme spelled out in the Act, perceiving them as a threat to doctors' autonomy. The OMA distributed pamphlets to doctors' offices and warned patients that if OMSIP paid doctors, '(you) might wake up some morning and find your doctor working for the government, not you'.[6] At the June OMA Annual Meeting, a resolution was approved to bill patients directly and sign contracts with Physicians Services Inc (private insurance) instead of OMSIP contracts (*The Globe and Mail*, 1966).

In April 1967, the OMA released its new fee schedule, which included increases of up to 30 per cent for some specialist fees. The increases were badly received by government. Minister Dymond appreciated, however, that 'emphasis (in the new schedule) has been placed on the need to increase fees for general practitioners',[7] although he also said he was 'determined to see that this will not happen again' (*Toronto Star*, 1967). Eventually, during that year, an agreement was reached between the government and the OMA regarding the fee negotiation process. Minister Dymond insisted that any future increase in doctors' fees be subject to negotiation (*Toronto Star*, 1968). Doctors claimed the OMA fee schedule was a guideline and they were free to charge what they wished.

An editorial in the *Toronto Star* emphasised that most doctors were cooperating with the OMSIP: 'In general, doctors are prospering under OMSIP' (Doig, 1967; OMSIP, 1967). In 1968, OMA President Dr Melvin came out harshly against the Medicare plan, objecting to the lack of consultation, and the 'communist' nature of the plan that went against the 'old-fashioned broad-based democratic ideals toward an often poorly informed central control'. Although he did say, 'I think we will accept it, and try to make it work … provided it's fair' (quoted in Millin, 1968). He made assurances that there was no intention to strike and 'that nobody really wins in strike' (quoted in Hollobon, 1968).

The Act respecting health services insurance (SO, 1969, c. 43) of 1969 represented the real introduction of full Ontario Medicare.[8] The Ontario Act stated that the schedule of fees could be revised by the OMA, but the Minister reserved the power to establish fees by regulation (Section 21). It did not prohibit extra billing by medical doctors and the Minister could make arrangements with doctors to pay them otherwise than by FFS. The Act also provided for a Medical Eligibility Committee composed only of doctors appointed by the Minister of Health to regulate physician payments.

Consolidating Ontario Medicare: managing turbulence, 1970–91

The 1970s saw Medicare take shape under the stable PC government of Bill Davis (1971–85). The tradition of selecting medical doctors as Ministers of Health in Ontario was broken after 1970, suggesting a decrease in medical control over the healthcare system to the advantage of the State and its bureaucrats (Coburn, 1993).[9]

The *Toronto Star* ran a special report on the first anniversary of Ontario Medicare. It found that doctors were gradually abandoning their demand for full payment of fees, with 60 per cent of them collecting the 90 per cent paid by the Medicare plan without charging patients the extra 10 per cent. Dr Glenn Sawyer, General Secretary of the OMA, said: 'our doctors are very much satisfied with OHSIP. We have the best care plan in Canada' (quoted in Malling, 1970).

In July 1971, the Ontario Legislature introduced Bill 5, the Health Insurance Organisation Act (Bill 5, 1971/SO, 1971, c. 5), which reduced the flexibility doctors had to bill both the Ontario Health Insurance Plan (OHIP) and patients. Doctors therefore had to decide whether to bill the OHIP and accept 90 per cent of the fee recommended by the OMA, or opt out of the plan and bill patients directly for the entire fee, and leave it to patients to request reimbursement of the OHIP fee amount (*Toronto Star*, 1971a). Health Minister Bert Lawrence told doctors 'government has no intention of telling doctors how to practise medicine but will make sure that every dollar they get from the OHSIP is legitimately earned' (*Toronto Star*, 1971a).

The OMA regarded the bill as 'harassment' and a challenge to medical doctors' autonomy. In an open letter to Ontario citizens, the OMA called on them to 'let the politicians of all political parties know that you want your personal medical services to remain a confidential matter between you and your doctor. And that politicians and civil servants have no place in the consulting rooms ... or on the doctors' backs' (*Toronto Star*, 1971b). The OMA advised its members to bypass the OHIP and to bill patients directly. There were also calls for the OMA to organise itself as a trade union and to hire tough negotiators to bargain with government (Dunlop, 1971).

In 1972, the Act respecting Health Insurance (Bill 184, 1972/SO, 1972, c. 91) enacted the OHIP and gave power over this plan to a general manager nominated by the Minister of Health. The Act again gave the OMA power to negotiate the schedule of fees with the Minister of Health (Section 31).

The Ministry of Health was also remodelled in 1972. Bill 185, Act respecting the Ministry of Health (Bill 185, 1972/SO, 1972, c. 92), stipulated that the Minister must enter into agreements with medical doctors in order to offer payment on a basis other than an FFS, which limited its power in this area (Dunlop, 1971, section 6(1)d).

The Health Disciplines Act (Bill 22, 1974/SO, 1974, c. 47) was introduced in February 1974, giving the Minister power to force the College of Physicians and Surgeons of Ontario (CPSO) to modify any regulations with a prior notice of 60 days.[10] In 1980, the Ontario College approved in principle a new system of peer checks on doctors' practices that extended the type of review conducted in hospitals through accreditation exercises to doctors in private practice. These reviews were educational rather than punitive, and doctors who needed to improve would be told to take a refresher course (Newbery, 1980).

During this period, Community Health Clinics (CHCs) were held out as having a major role to play in 'providing primary health care in the province in the next 10 years' (*Toronto Star*, 1972). Health Service Organisations (HSOs) were also being established in some communities. This 'increased fears of many doctors that CHCs would replace the traditional method of providing care in doctors' offices and make the solo practitioner archaic' (*Toronto Star*, 1972). The focus on CHCs drew on a report by a committee headed by Dr John Hastings of the University of Toronto. Dr Sawyer from the OMA proposed conducting pilot projects, with OMA assistance, and evaluating them before moving further ahead (Dunlop, 1972a). The model gained favour from the CMA, Canadian Hospital Association and Canadian Nurses' Association, which passed a joint resolution to expand community clinics to fill healthcare gaps and expand nurses' responsibilities (Dunlop, 1972b). Aggarwal considers the experience with HSOs to exemplify government's 'accommodative relationship with the medical association', with government diluting the initial design of the model due to the resistance from the OMA and other groups (Aggarwal, 2009: 116, 118–19). In 1975, Health Minister Frank Miller 'put a halt to further expansion of CHCs and HSOs, citing the OMA position that there was inadequate evidence and evaluation of their effectiveness' (quoted in Aggarwal, 2009: 119).

Between 1970 and 1978, OHIP claims increased from $32 million to $56 million per year. In 1976, doctor fees were increased 8.1 per cent in an agreement negotiated between the OMA and government. Two oil crises and rising inflation prompted the introduction of wage and price controls across Canada in the second half of the decade, tempering any increase in doctors' fees. Ontario's Health Minister planned to close 3,000 general hospital beds across the province. The OMA deplored the decisions that did not seem to be based on evidence or consultation with healthcare organisations (CMA, 1976).

In 1978, Ontario's government changed the rules governing the setting of fees. The government – working with the OMA – established its own fee schedule, which was 30 per cent below the OMA schedule. The decision to unhitch OHIP benefits from the OMA fee schedule would soon be seen as the turning point to souring relations between government and the medical profession (Dunlop, 1980). It starkly revealed the gap between what doctors thought their services were worth and what government was willing to pay. In the six months to April 1979, the percentage of doctors opting out and billing patients directly (and often above OHIP rates) increased from 13 per cent to nearly 18 per cent (Weiers, 1979). Opting out became the doctor version of strikes and placards (Weiers, 1979). Federal Health Minister Monique Bégin expressed concern about the number of doctors across the country opting out of Medicare and about the amount patients were being charged over and above insured levels. She raised the threat of holding back federal contributions (Heller, 1979), but also encouraged provinces to compensate doctors fairly. 'We feel the doctors didn't get a good deal on the latest round of schedules', she told the *Toronto Star* in March 1979 (Henderich, 1979).

Health Minister Dennis Timbrell negotiated with the OMA to restore a spirit of cooperation in 1979. He recognised that doctors had a right to opt out, that the principle of self-regulation had to be maintained and that doctors should be fairly paid and have the right to extra bill (Manthorpe, 1979). The OMA achieved an 11.5 per cent increase in its overall envelope from OHIP over 1979–80 (*Toronto Star*, 1980). Jonathan Manthorpe of the *Toronto Star* commented the dynamic emerging in the 1979 negotiations:

> The government has been most tender in putting the boot to the OMA. One cannot imagine the Tories dealing with any other trade union, with the possible exception of the Law Society of Upper

Canada, with such deference ... we see here in Timbrell's statement the beginnings of the notion that a union with a closed shop, with a monopoly, has only limited rights in industrial action, which is what the opting-out epidemic has been. Doctors as individuals have every right to drop out of the Medicare system, but doctors as a community have the obligation to make sure that does not endanger OHIP. (Manthorpe, 1979)

In the 1980s, Health Minister Larry Grossman, in the position for just a year and a half (1982–83), took an interest in CHCs and HSOs and convened a task force under Dr Fraser Mustard (Aggarwal, 2009: 119). The Mustard Report recommended wide expansion of HSOs and the implementation of CHCs. While government supported the recommendation, the expansion was voluntary and the OMA warned doctors against propagating state-controlled healthcare: '(B)etween 1979 and 1987, HSOs grew from 13 to only 27 primary care organisations' (Aggarwal, 2009: 121; Gillett et al, 2001).

Fee negotiations between the OMA and government in 1981 were coloured by the 30 per cent gap between OMA fees and OHIP rates, coupled with the federal government's desire to ban extra charges (which amounted to some $3.2 billion in Ontario) (Haliechuk, 1981). The OMA Council rejected the government's offer of a 14.75 per cent increase, despite it being supported by the Health Minister and the President of the OMA. At the start of 1982, the OMA was encouraging doctors to close their offices for one day, followed by rotating walkouts to pressure government to increase fees by 31.2 per cent along with cost of living adjustments. The generous increase other provinces had negotiated in 1981 meant that Ontario doctors had gone from being the best paid in the country to 10 per cent below average (Gordon and Dunlop, 1982). At an OMA assembly, Dr Moran told the 1,000 doctors assembled: 'The greatest single threat to health care in Ontario is the government. And the OMA has a public responsibility to maintain the balance of power in determining the level of care that will be delivered.' The government and the OMA finally reached a settlement in May 1982, giving doctors a 41 per cent increase in fees over the next three years (Crowe, 1982).

In 1984, when the federal government adopted the CHA prohibiting extra billing and user charges, the OMA instituted a legal challenge (CMA, 1984) against the constitutionality of the law. The OMA urged doctors to support a right-wing National Citizens' Coalition – founded in 1967 by an insurance salesman – to fight the CHA. Ontario Health Minister Keith Norton said he would not rule out any option on extra billing and that government was studying the 'most appropriate' mechanism for complying with the Act (Crawford, 1984).

The Ontario election was called for May 1985. Election results saw the PCs win 52 seats, Liberals 48 and the New Democratic Party (NDP) 25. In

May 1985, the Ontario Liberals struck a deal with the NDP for its support over at least two years; the NDP's conditions were government action to expand rent control and ban extra billing (Harrington, 1985a).

After the Liberals took power, Dr Michael Rachlis, Head of the Medical Reform Group (MRG) that defended the public system and stood against extra billing, said 'I think we can expect a really messy, hardball campaign with walkouts in certain localities' (quoted in Flavelle, 1985). He supported negotiating a settlement between doctors and government that would increase fees in exchange for a ban on extra billing. Bill 94, introduced in Ontario legislature in December, imposed substantial fines on doctors if they charged patients more than Medicare rates. OMA President Dr Myers said the Bill left Ontario doctors worse off than those in Québec, who at least had the option of opting out entirely (Dunlop and Newbery, 1985). The OMA Board decided to ask its 17,000 members to again withdraw services, close offices and cancel non-urgent surgeries, in order to fight the ban on extra billing.

Meanwhile, the federal government was holding on to some $50 million in withheld transfer payments, and the province had until 1987 to apply the CHA.

In 1986, OMA chair and chief negotiator Dr Hugh Scully called for the 'strongest possible measures' to preserve extra billing (Deverell, 1986). The OMA considered the act an oppressive use of government power that would deny physicians the right to make a simple contract with a patient. Another suit was launched against Bill 94, considered in violation of the Canadian Charter (Harrington, 1985b; Newbery, 1986). Pressure tactics were supported by the majority of medical doctors and culminated in an indefinite strike in June that would last 25 days, making it the longest strike in Canada after the introduction of Medicare.

However, the OMA was out of step with public mood. At a news conference in March 1986, Judy Rebick spoke for a coalition of 40 unions when she stated: 'It's a fight between the doctors and the people of Ontario' (quoted in Harrington, 1986). There was also division within the medical community: the MRG provided an effective counter-narrative to the OMA position. Spokesperson Dr Trevor Hancock stated: 'extra-billing is the single greatest threat to a truly accessible health system'; he considered that many doctors were 'too intimidated' to oppose the OMA, whose leaders 'are leading the doctors in a fight they can't possibly win' (quoted in J. Ferguson, 1986).

Bill 94 was adopted in June. By July, more and more doctors were re-establishing normal services and the strike was called off. OMA President Dr Richard Railton recognised Premier Peterson had little choice, under pressure from both the NDP and federal penalties, but also that doctors had failed to persuade the public. University of Toronto political economist, John

Crispo, considered: 'The doctors emerged from the strike with nothing to show for their efforts except a cruel lesson in humility' (quoted in R. Ferguson, 1986).

Bill 94 also introduced ideas about changing the status of the OMA to have it recognised as sole bargaining agent for Ontario doctors in fee negotiations with the government.[11] While this would entitle the OMA to mediation, it would also mean that a full member vote would be needed to call a strike, reducing the power of the 250-member governing Council.

For Carolyn Tuohy, the 1986 doctor's strike stood out as the only one 'in which such tactics failed to win substantial concessions from the state in Canada' (Tuohy, 1988, note 267).[12] It represented a brief 'episode of conflict in a long history of accommodation between medicine and the state' (Tuohy, 1988: 270). Indeed, the government's victory in this all-important battle made it more conciliatory during 1987 negotiations over the OHIP fee schedule.

Following the ban on extra billing, a steep increase of 17 per cent in 1987 in the total amount doctors billed focused attention on the FFS payment mechanism and heightened the perception of out-of-control spending in health. In opposition, the NDP highlighted alternatives and the MRG supported moving away from FFS, presenting capitation as a more suitable system for family physicians.

At the end of 1987, Peterson created the Premier's Council on Health to develop a long-term strategy for healthcare. The Council included the new Minister of Health, Elinor Caplan, along with representatives from business, labour, healthcare and the public. In explaining the Council's goals, Peterson said 'We will be moving toward a community-based system, rather than just an institutional system' (quoted in Milnes and Zade, 2017). With regard to medical doctors' billing, the Council looked with interest at fee caps introduced in both Québec and BC. In December 1988, the government imposed a settlement on doctors for the first time, raising fees by 1.75 per cent, and not the 5.7 per cent demanded by the OMA (*Toronto Star*, 1989).

In 1989, the Liberal government passed the Act respecting independent health facilities (Bill 147, 1989/SO, 1989, c. 59) to regulate the expansion of healthcare facilities outside of hospitals, such as ambulatory diagnostic and treatment clinics (Coburn et al, 1997). Consultations on the Bill lasted for over a year and affected 1,800 existing facilities. The OMA described it as 'draconian legislation … which will provide for far-reaching bureaucratic control under the guise of funding new services' (quoted in Wyman, 1989: 203).

Heading into new fee negotiations in 1990, the OMA was eager to avoid the risk of repeating an imposed deal. The Council adopted a Position Paper proposed by the OMA Board called *Toward a Partnership in the 1990s* (Sullivan, 1990), which aimed to achieve binding arbitration around negotiation of the OHIP fee schedule. In June 1990, the OMA decided to stop the court actions against the CHA and Bill 94.

Once in office after elections in October 1990, Bob Rae's NDP and Health Minister Frances Lankin set out to shift spending from institutions to community services. The NDP introduced the Regulated Health Professions Act (Bill 43, SO, 1991, c. 18), along with 21 'companion' bills (44–64) that addressed the regulation of 24 different health professions and aimed to give the public 'a louder and clearer voice than they ever had in how the healthcare system operates'.[13]

A companion bill, the Medicine Act (Bill 55 – SO 1991, c. 30) addressed medical doctors. The OMA indicated being 'supportive of the legislation', especially the creation of a 'quality assurance committee'.[14] However, it demanded the reintegration of a 'harm clause' in the list of controlled acts, which would increase their number. The CPSO also demanded the return of the 'harm clause' in the final law and a maximum ratio of 40 per cent of public members on its council,[15] and denounced the increased direct power of the Health Minister over the College.

In the Regulated Health Professions Act as adopted (SO, 1991, c. 18), the 'harm clause' was reinstated (section 30) and the final Bill also obliged the minister to give 30 days' notice to all members of the Council before imposing regulations on the College (sections 10(2)), which better protected the College's autonomy.

Finally, OMA negotiations with government in spring 1991 took place in the context of a larger Framework Agreement that sought to establish longer-term stability. The Ontario Medical Association Dues Act (Bill 135, SO, 1991, c. 51)[16] required that all doctors pay dues to the OMA, regardless of whether they joined as members;[17] [18] it also included a binding arbitration clause and finally confirmed the OMA as the only bargaining representative of all Ontario medical doctors 'in matters affecting both fee-for-service and non-fee-for-service'.[19] 'Finally, the agreement establishe[d] a Joint Management Committee (JMC), which gave both the OMA and the government a voice in determining the future direction of health care in Ontario' (Goldman, 1991; Tenszen, 1991). The agreement went to a member vote and was overwhelmingly approved.

The OMA gained 'veto power over the allocation of funding for physician services [which] meant that the government could not redistribute FFS funding to alternative service delivery without the approval of the OMA' (Aggarwal, 2009: 81).

Recession hits: restructuring through the social contract and the 'Common Sense Revolution', 1991–96

The fragile equilibrium achieved between medical doctors and the government rapidly shattered later in 1991 when the province entered its worst recession since the early 1980s. Spending cuts by both federal and provincial governments, coupled with a Bank of Canada increase in interest rates, acted as a drag on the economy that prolonged the recession into 1996–97 (Mckenzi, 2010). At the end of 1991, Health Minister Frances Lankin said: 'Ontario simply can't afford its present healthcare system' (quoted in Priest, 1992). The government proposed the Social Contract Act in June 1993, imposing a three-year wage freeze and allowing for a forced 12 days' unpaid leave for all civil service workers who earned more than $30,000 per year (Hebdon and Warrian, 1999).

Less than a year after concluding the long-term agreement with the OMA, Minister Lankin sought to renegotiate it to adapt to the new economic reality. The government introduced Bill 50 (Expenditure Control Plan Statute Law Amendment Act) that gave it the power to control access to medical services (Walkom, 1993). The aim was to cut $1 billion from the health budget. In negotiations with the OMA, the government had a number of advantages. First, the number of doctors in Ontario had grown by 47 per cent between 1975 and 1990, while the population had increased by just 19 per cent, and other provinces had taken measures earlier to reduce the number of doctors (Priest, 1993a). Second, the public and government were largely unsympathetic to doctors' complaints around fees as many households were devastated by long recession (Priest, 1993b).

In the Interim Agreement of Economic Arrangements of August 1993, the government imposed a 'hard cap' (Priest, 1993c) cutting the total funding envelope going to Ontario doctors by 5.5 per cent, and seeking to save $20 million by delisting some procedures and limiting coverage of others. When total billings were found to exceed the cap before the end of the year, the more progressive OMA Board recommended that OHIP hold back 4.8 per cent of payments to medical doctors (CMA, 1993). There appeared to be some dissent, however, within the OMA (and more broadly among doctors) about their duty to help reduce costs without putting patient care at risk.

Bill 50 allowed the government to suspend its contractual obligations with health services providers on the matters of agreed payments and related negotiation, mediation or arbitration, until 1 April 1996.[20] Towards the end of 1994, doctors were discouraging patients from booking appointments for minor problems, reminding them that they were working 'for free', and the Ministry was supportive of this approach (Priest, 1994a). Billings were more than $200 million over the hard cap, double what doctors had had to 'pay back' in 1993–94 (Priest, 1994b). In February 1995, OMA representatives turned their backs on the Joint Management Committee because the government unilaterally decided to impose a general percentage.

A reinvigorated PC party under Mike Harris launched its 'Common Sense Revolution' platform in May 1994, detailing an approach to deficit cutting. The 'common sense' message earned the PCs 49 per cent of the vote in June 1995 elections, with many appreciating Harris' 'realism' despite its hard edge (Bradburn, 2018).

In healthcare, the government wanted 'to assist hospitals to restructure further' by establishing a Health Services Restructuring Commission (HSRC) led by Dr Duncan Sinclair, former Dean of Medicine at Queen's University, to manage and accelerate the implementation of reforms. The government also announced it would 'take steps to address longstanding problems with the delivery of physicians' services. We will ensure a fair distribution of doctors between urban and rural areas'.[21]

Bill 26 (Savings and Restructuring Act) increased the Minister of Health's powers over public hospital organisations, including the power to close hospitals in consideration of public interest. Bill 26 gave doctors very little recourse if their hospital was chosen for closure or consolidation; appeals regarding hospital privileges would be limited. Privileges could be revoked without input from medical advisory committees or hospital boards once the board or Health Minister decided the hospital should close (*Medical Post*, 1996e). Schedule I of Bill 26, the Physician Services Delivery Management Act, 'terminated all previous agreements with the OMA [and] eliminated its exclusive right to represent the profession in negotiations with government' (Flood and Erdman, 2004).

Medical doctors were challenged to find new ways to respond to the government's power play. At the start of 1996, the OMA opted for media campaigns, education and communication rather than strike action to express opposition to restructuring plans. Trying to dispel a reputation as 'obstructionist' and pave the way to collaborative relations during the Tories' term, the OMA was civil in its critique of Bill 26, while still expressing its concerns (*Medical Post*, 1996e).

In an interview conducted during public hearings on Bill 26, Health Minister Jim Wilson stated: 'We don't want an agreement with binding arbitration. ... Neither the 1991 nor 1993 agreements have served the public or physicians very well' (*Medical Post*, 1996a). He considered it unhelpful for the OMA to have exclusive representation rights. In response, OMA President Dr Bill Orovan argued that the OMA was essential to protecting the livelihoods of doctors and having a say in the management of the health system, especially as alternate payment plans (APPs) were now going to be coming from the FFS pool (MedPost, 1996b: 22–3).

In January 1996, the omnibus Bill 26 was passed, giving the government new powers to set medical doctors' fees, determine what services were medically necessary, access information in patient charts, and determine where medical doctors could practise (*Medical Post*, 1996c). After objections expressed by the OMA, the government amended the bill to put a time limit on the extraordinary powers for hospital restructuring.[22]

Minister Wilson expressed openness to new ways of working with doctors and a number of more collaborative initiatives were begun in this environment. Most significant was new medical doctors' interest in non-FFS payment schemes such as capitation, as doctors anticipated large spending cuts. However, doctors insisted they must be 'in the loop' in planning the model (*Medical Post*, 1996d).

Primary care reform, 1996–2004

An early collaborative development between medical doctors and the government was the invigoration of primary care reform, led from 1996 by Dr Wendy Graham, chair of the OMA's Primary Care Reform Physician Advisory Group, and supported by Minister Wilson. The Group presented a discussion paper, *Primary Care Reform: A Strategy for Stability*, on ways to change 'how the province's 10,000 family physicians get paid, deliver care and where they work' (quoted in Priest, 1996). The proposal called for patients to sign contracts with doctors to cut down on 'doctor shopping', rostering, and payment through modified FFS (part FFS, part based on a panel of patients in order to deter overuse of tests and treatments; see Priest, 1996; Tuohy 1999: 223; Aggarwal, 2009: 137). The proposal was seen by the OMA as an 'antidote' to Bill 26 that sought to restrict where doctors could practise by limited billing numbers. It would provide a better way of assuring adequate distribution by having patients enrol with a given medical doctor or group and paying doctors through capitation: a dollar amount per enrolled patient (Tuohy, 1999: 223; Aggarwal, 2009: 137).

The OMA endorsed the discussion paper and creation of primary care groups, eventually called Primary Care Networks (PCNs). Opposition to primary care reform was rooted in concern to preserve autonomy, freedom of choice in practice model and a distaste for managed care (Richardson, 1997).

PCNs were similar to HSOs: 'The difference between these models was that the PCN model consisted of a blended model of capitation and FFS in which there were more FFS incentives' (Aggarwal, 2009: 141). Lazar et al, in their book *Paradigm Freeze*, state that 'significant numbers of [primary care] physicians [are] now practicing under the terms of formal contracts with the Ministry of Health and Long-Term Care and under a blended payment mechanism, which has altered the traditional, public FFS payment mechanism in use for more than three decades' (Lazar et al, 2013). Tuohy considers it relevant that the government 'appointed the family physician who had chaired the OMA Primary Care Reform Advisory Group to chair an implementation steering committee' (Tuohy, 1999: 223) for PCNs.

It would take until December 1997 for new Health Minister, Elizabeth Witmer, to announce the province would go ahead with the pilot projects in primary care. Sinclair, of the HSRC, urged the government to introduce changes quickly: 'The time for pilots is past ... it is time for the Big Bang.

I think we should just do primary care reform and do it everywhere, all at once, and soon' (Muncin, 1997).

Support for primary care reforms from OMA members was strong, at 75 per cent among GPs and 80 per cent among specialists (Borsellino, 1998a).

The Coalition of Family Physicians of Ontario, created in 1996, stepped up efforts to gain strength within the OMA, assembling funds and structures to participate in debate around primary care reform (*Medical Post*, 1997). It also campaigned to see the OMA stripped of its role as the profession's exclusive bargaining agent, which had been granted in 1991, threatened during 1996 negotiations, and reinstated in the final 1997 Agreement. Pilot sites were announced in June 1998, a full two years after the OMA had unveiled its plan (Borsellino, 1998b).

In February 1998, the government passed the Expanded Nursing Services for Patients Act (Bill 127, 1997/SO, 1997, c. 9). The OMA was involved in consultations and was satisfied with the legislation, although remained concerned around independent practice and how nurse practitioners (NPs) would be paid (Wansbrough, 1998). OMA President Dr Albert Schumacher saw a role for NPs in PCNs, where an NP would allow 800 extra patients to be enrolled (Borsellino, 2000).

The quality and accountability reform agenda, 2000–09

By 2000, demands for increased accountability and quality were evident in healthcare systems across Canada (Baker et al, 2004; Dobrow, Goel, and Lemieux-Charles, 2006). Ontario was also facing a wait times crisis for cancer treatments, with a significant number of patients being sent to the US for treatment (OBHC, JL, at 10). Wait times were considered a threat to the acceptability of Medicare. Federal Minister Paul Martin announced the 'deal for a decade', increasing federal transfers to the provinces, with some strings attached. Martin singled out wait times as the key barometer for Canadians' satisfaction with healthcare and agreed to set national benchmarks for medically acceptable wait times in five areas, including cancer and advanced diagnostics (Pole, 2004).

The Ontario Liberals under Dalton McGuinty won by a landslide on a platform to roll back tax breaks and reinvest in schools and hospitals (Demont, 2003). The new government immediately set to assure Ontarians of their 'total commitment' to Medicare.

Health Minister Smitherman introduced Bill 8, the Commitment to the Future of Medicare Act. Citing the federal Romanow report, which proposed that accountability be added as a fundamental of Canadian Medicare, he promised Bill 8 would entrench accountability as a cornerstone in Ontario.[23] Bill 8 required that medical doctors deal directly with the OHIP, eliminating the right to opt out of Medicare, and it imposed accountability agreements

(Borsellino, 2003). Smitherman said he was open to advice on the Bill (Borsellino, 2004a). The OMA obtained a number of amendments: medical doctors would be exempt from accountability provisions; restructuring of various payment mechanisms, including sessional payments, were lifted, as was Ministry (and OHIP) power to collect, use and disclose personal information about patients and physicians 'for any purpose they prescribe'; and penalties for extra billing no longer included jail time and maximum fines were significantly reduced (Borsellino, 2004b).

Dr Alan Hudson joined the government's Health Results team led by Dr Hugh McLeod to spread the Liberal government's health transformation agenda and communicate expected behaviour changes from specialists in hospitals to track and reduce wait times: 'No one in Ontario has really been accountable for making sure patients have appropriate access', he said (quoted in Borsellino, 2005e). 'Our strategy makes hospital boards accountable for equitable access in their organisations' (Borsellino, 2005e). Hudson took a hard line with doctors: 'My advice to [physicians] is to realise the world is changing very quickly. They should start working with the public and administrators and politicians to help shape the future. The days of any surgical group determining what's going to happen are over' (Borsellino, 2005d).

The OMA was also negotiating a service agreement with the Ministry over the first nine months of 2004 that included extensive fee adjustments, including a new comprehensive care management fee for primary care medical doctors. The deal found unanimous support from the OMA negotiating team, but the OMA Council wanted member endorsement (Borsellino, 2004c). In November 2004, the Specialist Coalition, Coalition of Family Physicians and Family Practice and General Practice (GP–FP) section of the OMA voted overwhelmingly to turn down the deal (Borsellino, 2004d). The Specialist Coalition considered it 'dictates how doctors practise medicine and treats doctors as government employees' (Borsellino, 2004d). Minister Smitherman released details of modifications made to respond to OMA concerns and considered imposing the deal on medical doctors. In this, he risked a potential violation of the Canada Health Act, which called for binding arbitration in case of impasse between doctors and government (Borsellino, 2004e). It would take several more months before the OMA Board unanimously endorsed the four-year deal. It awarded more generous retroactive fee increases, eliminated billing thresholds, allowed doctors to incorporate, and got rid of incentives to medical doctors to keep drug costs down, along with earlier concessions (Borsellino, 2005a, b; Cary, 2005; Ferguson, 2005).

The other issue coming to the fore was the audit process used to verify medical doctors' billings. Supreme Court Justice Peter Cory was conducting a Medical Audit Practice Review to inform changes to the process (deCarteret

Cory, 2005). Reforming the audit process became a key priority for the OMA (Borsellino, 2005c). The government introduced the Transitional Physician Payment Review Act (Bill 104, 2004) that put in place a transitional board to review physician billings (the Transitional Physician Audit Panel) in place of the former Medical Review Committee.[24] Justice Cory released his final report in April 2005 (Cory, 2005), in which he was very critical of the previous medical audit system[25] (as was the OMA), and proposed 118 recommendations to create a new and improved regulatory system. Many of his recommendations were implemented in the 2006 Bill 171, the Health System Improvements Act.

As negotiations with the OMA continued into 2005, the Ministry unveiled yet another model for primary care. Family Health Teams would have a board of directors that followed a governance and accountability roadmap, various health professionals working as a cooperative team, appropriate office infrastructure and a clinical management system built around an electronic health record (EHR). Dr Garnet Maley, who helped design the Family Health Group model, was named chair of the OMA section on group practice, which had been largely 'dormant'.

The Health System Improvement Act (Bill 171) modified the powers of the OHIP general manager and established the Physician Payment Review Board.[26] This was composed of between 20 and 30 medical doctors, half of whom were selected by the OMA, and six to 10 members of the public.[27] It functioned as a quasi-judicial body to determinate if a medical doctor's billing was appropriate. OMA President, Dr Janice Willett, called the new audit system 'a big improvement' (quoted in Kondro, 2007).

In 2009, Health Minister Deb Matthews introduced the Regulated Health Professions Statute Law Amendment Act (Bill 179, 2009/SO, 2009, c. 26), which aimed to increase accessibility and quality of care by authorising some health professionals such as midwives, dentists, dental hygienists, NPs and pharmacists to perform additional regulated acts independently from medical doctors: 'The Ontario Medical Association responded with full-page newspaper ads warning Ontarians that [their] health is at stake. ... Ontario Hospital Association CEO Tom Closson alleged in the Star that the OMA's opposition to Bill 179 exemplified its pattern of turf protection' (Rachlis, 2009).

OMA President Dr Suzanne Strasberg indicated that 'Bill 179 contains a number of recommendations that reflect positions brought forward by [the OMA]. The OMA's submission to the Standing Committee expressed concern with the lack of oversight by medical doctors of NPs and pharmacists for the new regulated medical acts' (OMA, 2009).[28]

In its submission to the committee (CPSO, 2009), the CPSO criticised the provisions in the Bill that would give the Minister the power to appoint a supervisor to take over all the functions of the College's councils.[29] The government stuck to its initial proposition, despite the OMA's media campaign against it, encouraged by other colleges, the OHA, and the popularity of the Bill's goals: better access to and sustainability of healthcare.

The quality and accountability agenda: a patient-oriented project, 2010–19

In 2010, the Liberals introduced the Excellent Care for All Act (Bill 46, 2010/SO, 2010, c. 14). Like the Commitment to the Future of Medicare Act 2004, these accountability measures did not apply to individual medical doctors or to primary care models. During parliamentary hearings, the OMA was supporting increased accountability of boards and administrators as well as 'the government's attempt to place patients and patient experience at the centre of the system' (Standing Committee on Justice Policy, 20 May 2010). The OMA also insisted on keeping quality evaluation in the hands of clinical leaders. The OMA asked during the hearings that a sufficient consultation period be given to medical doctors before fully implementing the regulations, considering the complexity of the legislation.

A joint effort by the Ontario Hospital Association (OHA), the Association of Community Care Access Centres and the Ontario Federation of Community Mental Health and Addiction programmes produced a report recommending ways to save $2 billion from Ontario's health budget (Borsellino, 2010b; Vogel, 2010). Part of that involved amending the Public Hospitals Act to move away from the current system of medical doctor privileges and towards a hospital–medical doctor contract model that could be used to specify terms of medical doctor reimbursement, provide hospitals greater flexibility to evaluate medical doctors on the basis of performance and quality, and assure that payment reflected the aims of hospitals.

The OHA introduced prototype bylaws that would move toward greater accountability. These were not well received by medical doctors, who saw them as a way to reduce their influence in hospital decision-making (Vogel, 2010). The new bylaws, introduced unilaterally by the OHA without traditional input from the OMA and Canadian Medical Protective Association (CMPA), also made medical doctors part of the hospital's 'professional staff', with positions needing approval of the CEO as well as the Medical Advisory Committee. The OHA was encouraging other hospitals to adopt the bylaws (Borsellino, 2010a). The CPSO gave its blessing to a plan for academic health centres to routinely assess all hospital credential-holding physicians. A pilot project was planned for 2011 using a model from the College of Physicians and Surgeons of Alberta (the Physician Achievement Review programme) (Sylvain, 2010).

In January 2012, the government released *Ontario's Action Plan for Health Care: Better Patient Care through Better Value from our Health Care Dollars*

(Ministry of Health and Long-Term Care [MOHLTC] – January 2012). The OMA assured doctors that 'The Action Plan shows no intent to transfer control of physician funding to the LHINs (Local Health Integration Networks, at regional governance level). In fact, the document states clearly that the role of physician funding will continue to reside with the ministry' (Belluz, 2012c).

In April 2012, the government began implementing Health System Funding Reform to transition from global funding to patient-based funding linked to volume and type of service. The reform was first applied to hospitals, Community Care Access Centres and long-term care centres. To allay medical doctors' fears about losing income, the Ministry incorporated funding risk mitigation measures, guaranteeing that their total income would not be far off levels in previous years (Kralj and Barber, 2013).

In parallel to these reform plans, in May 2011, the OMA was putting its negotiating team together in anticipation of talks to replace the current four-year deal that was set to expire in March 2012. With the provincial economy still fragile after the 2009 crash and the government calling for a freeze in public service-related contracts, the OMA said it would look for a fair settlement (Sylvain, 2011a, b). Besides, as *Medical Post* editor Colin Leslie considered, many at the OMA were thinking about how to prepare medicine for huge changes in accountability (Leslie, 2013b).

Negotiations with the OMA began with the government presenting a 'white binder' detailing its fiscal position and the increase in medical doctors' compensation over the past 15 years (Leslie, 2013a) and demanding $1 billion in cuts to fees and programmes over four years as a take-it-or-leave-it proposition. The OMA countered by offering a two-year freeze in fees, which the government rejected and then refused to continue negotiating with a third party conciliator. Minister Deb Matthews, in an interview with the *Toronto Star*, said medical doctors weren't considering the province's fiscal realities and the massive amount the province spent on doctors' fees (Koul, 2012).

In late May 2012, the government announced that it would make the unprecedented move of imposing unilateral cuts to doctors' fee schedules, the result of a regulatory change passed under the Health Insurance Act. The CMA threw its support behind OMA opposition because, in their opinion, Ontario's approach to bargaining flew in the face of the Canada Health Act, which states that governments have a duty to negotiate responsibly with medical doctors. 'If that kind of legislated approach to (negotiations) takes root across the country', warned CMA President Dr John Haggie, 'it'll be a game-changer. It'll wipe out the ability of doctors to negotiate' (quoted in Belluz, 2012a). The OMA launched a Charter challenge against the government (Belluz, 2012b).

Minister Matthews came back with an offer that was much more acceptable to the OMA. The OMA urged members to ratify the agreement, which 81 per cent of its members did (Belluz, 2012b): 'The two parties said the deal paves the way for smoother negotiations in the future, since it formalises the partnership between the government and the OMA and puts in place a conciliation process for future conflicts along the way' (Belluz, 2012b).

The 2012 Physician Services Agreement expired in March 2014. Minister of Health, Dr Eric Hoskins, asserted there would be no new funding for public sector employees, including medical doctors. After making no progress by September, Dr David Naylor was appointed facilitator (as per the 2012 Agreement), but no progress was achieved. Again, in line with the Agreement worked out in 2012, Chief Justice of Ontario Warren Winkler was brought in to assist in resolving outstanding issues. In 2015, the OMA Board formally rejected the offer and Minister Hoskins announced a 2.65 per cent cut to all FFS physician payments (Leslie, 2015a), restricted entry into Family Health Organisations (FHOs) and Family Health Networks (FHNs), discontinued enrolment premiums for healthy patients, and restricted the Income Stabilization programme (Harrison and Guo, 2015; see also Grant, 2015). The OMA indicated The OMA indicated that the economic situation is improving in Ontario and the government should reivest in healthcare and go back to the negotiation table with doctors (Leslie, 2015b). The government refused and made further cutbacks, reducing medical doctors' fees by another 1.3 per cent.[30] The OMA responded by launching a massive social media campaign. Made public, conciliator Winkler's report recommended that the government stand behind its offer and that the OMA reconsider rejecting it. He proposed a task force to recommend changes to the delivery and funding of physician services (Bronca, 2015).

Later in 2015, the OMA filed a Canadian Charter challenge against the Government of Ontario in the Superior Court. This aimed to establish mediation and binding arbitration mechanisms in the negotiation process (Leslie, 2016). The government was concerned that arbitrators did not always consider the taxpayer's ability to pay in their decisions (Leslie, 2016).

Following the government's unilateral actions, a group calling themselves Concerned Ontario Doctors came to life, organising a rally of doctors and patients in Queen's Park that recalled the 1986 doctors' strike (Bronca, 2016b).

When the government and the OMA Council arrived with a proposed Physician Services Agreement in 2016, some doctors received it as a shock after two years of acrimony. There was deep mistrust for the negotiating process (Alam, 2016). On the other hand, OMA President Dr Virginia Walley felt the contract gave the government and doctors a chance to work out details over time, with co-management mechanisms like the Physician Services Committee and the Medical Services Payment Committee. She said the prospects if the deal were rejected looked 'pretty grim'. 'We'll be in a position where we're not working together with government' (quoted in Anonymous, 2016).

The government then introduced an Act to amend various Acts in the interest of patient-centred care (Bill 41, 2016/SO, 2016, c. 30), or the Patients First Act 2016. In his presentation to the Standing Committee on Bill 41, OMA President-elect Dr Stephen Chris called the bill 'deeply disturbing to Ontario's doctors', notably because the government 'developed this plan without the expert advice from the family physicians'.[31] The OMA opposed making professional advisory committees optional and replacing them with patient and family advisory committees. The OMA considered that LHINs' power over human resources planning was in breach of the OMA's Representation Rights Agreement, as LHINs instead of government could regulate where medical doctors could work. The OMA considered that the government had an obligation to negotiate matters relating to medical doctor services and associated responsibilities with the OMA. Members of DoctorsOntario[32] and Concerned Ontario Doctors presented their objections to the Patients First Act, mainly that it added bureaucracy rather than services.[33] Concerned Ontario Doctors concluded by presenting the Committee with a petition signed by 21,000 Ontarians as a result of the #STOPBILL41 campaign.[34]

The OMA worked hard to gain support for the Agreement, which, importantly, struck out sections of the Patients First Act that would have given LHINs significant oversight over medical doctors. Supporters of the Agreement included a broad coalition of healthcare organisations and some sections of the OMA. Opponents were the Coalition of Ontario Doctors, Doctors Ontario and some OMA specialty sections. They forced the OMA to hold a binding vote and the Agreement was defeated (Boyle, 2016a, 2017a).

The Coalition had campaigned against this Agreement and more globally against the OMA's monopoly over medical doctor representation.[35] In a suit against OMA leadership brought by the Coalition before the vote, a Superior Court judge instructed the OMA leaders not to re-enter negotiations without binding arbitration, and to keep OMA sections fully apprised (Bronca, 2016c).

Later in August, Minister Hoskins said the government was open to recognising the OMA as a public sector union, but that would mean doctors' earnings would be made public and they would lose the tax advantage of being allowed to incorporate individually (Boyle, 2016b). The Coalition made its political views clear, hoping for a PC victory in elections (Boyle, 2016a). Hundreds of doctors then signed an open letter entitled 'A way forward for Ontario's doctors: Shared principles', which proposed embracing the OMA as the unified voice of the profession; fair and binding arbitration; medical doctor acceptance of their responsibility to maximise value;

commitment to address pay imbalances among doctors; and commitment to the principle of equity (Bronca, 2016d).

At the start of 2017, the Coalition of Ontario Doctors staged what some called a 'coup' to overthrow the OMA's executive committee (Boyle, 2017a). A no-confidence vote passed by 55 per cent, and a week later the executive of the OMA collectively resigned, although they remained on the Board (Boyle, 2017b).

In the lead-up to 2018 elections, the OMA produced an ad campaign, 'Not a second longer', aimed at putting pressure on candidates to reduce wait times.[36] Some of the ads stated: 'It's the government that keeps you waiting' and 'This election make your health matter.' The OMA also organised healthcare debates between candidates, which liberal candidates did not always attend. The OMA advocated against forcing doctors to spend more of their time dealing with bureaucrats and in favour of better integrating physicians in the planning and implementation of reforms.[37]

Concerned Ontario Doctors campaigned against the re-election of the Liberal Party and the OMA monopoly over medical doctors' representation (#CareNotCuts and #ExposeOMA).[38]

Elections on 7 June 2018 saw the end of 15 years of Liberal government and the election of the PCs under Premier Doug Ford. Ontario medical doctors had been without an agreement on fees since 2014. In February 2019, three arbitrators reached what the OMA and Ministry both called a sensible compromise. It did not undo all the cuts to physician payments over the years, but was satisfactory (Bronca, 2019).

The Premier's Council on Improving Healthcare and Ending Hallway Medicine produced recommendations for improving the integration of services. In 2019, Health Minister Christine Elliott introduced the People's Health Care Act, designed to make healthcare 'seamless'. OHA President Anthony Dale applauded the direction: 'What the minister's doing today is basically lifting some of that inappropriate oversight and red tape and third party intermediaries that get in the way of care providers actually working together', he said.

Part 4: Analysis of the Ontario case

The inception of Ontario Medicare: reconciling expectations, 1956–69

The influence of context: drivers and shapers of medical politics

A constellation of forces created intense health policy activity during this early period. In the 1950s, the Ontario government was busy getting organised and equipped to discuss healthcare reform, especially with the federal government, which expected a response to its call for better publicly funded coverage of care. To prepare, the Ontario government engaged in intense negotiations with the medical profession, hearing their multiple demands. Medical doctors wanted to be able to join the public insurance programme voluntarily and maintain control over their fees. The government also had to assess the acceptability to its political constituencies, including private insurance companies, of creating a publicly funded healthcare system. The creation of an agency like the Ontario Hospital Services Commission was emblematic of the government's determination to design a distinctly Ontarian version of Medicare. The government's initial preoccupation was with coverage for hospital care and finding options that would preserve a key role for private insurance companies within the healthcare system.

Strategies used to accommodate and deal with the evolving context

In the early 1960s, the OMA agreed to engage in negotiations with the government around the Medical Services Insurance Act (Holloran, 1990: 59). Ontario's Premier recognised that the voluntary public insurance programme advocated by the OMA would not meet universality criteria for federal funding. In early 1966, Premier Robarts pushed through legislation despite OMA resistance (Harold Greer, 'Ontario Medicare now law', 18 February 1966; and 'Ontario yields on Medicare, accepts compulsory coverage', *Toronto Star*, 26 October). The federal criteria provided government with considerable leverage as the importance of gaining access to the federal money on offer for healthcare was obvious. The OMA objected to any attempt by government to bypass the association and negotiate compensation policies directly with the medical profession, asserting that the OMA fee schedule was not open to negotiation with anybody (*Toronto Star*, 1966a). For the medical profession, the OMA's role was key to their professional autonomy and the principle of self-regulation. Through the OMA, medical doctors resisted government incursions using tactics such as press releases, petitions and the promotion of billing strategies that sidestepped the public plan. While the OMA opposed what they perceived as socialised medicine (Millin, 1968), most medical doctors embarked on the emerging public regime during this period and saw that their economic interests were protected when government paid the bill for medical services. After various proposals and amendments, the Act respecting health services insurance (SO, 1969, c. 43) was adopted in 1969 and stipulated that the new regime would cover 90 per cent of the costs of medical services and maintain the right for physicians to bill patients directly for the other 10 per cent. In its negotiations with the medical profession, the government referred to the more collaborative behaviours of medical doctors in other provinces.

Impact on medical politics and healthcare reforms

This initial stage in the emergence of a publicly funded healthcare system in Ontario was crucial in setting the tone for medical politics in the province. The government was able to secure a deal with a reluctant medical profession, but it left some issues unresolved, such as the right for medical doctors to engage in extra billing. This period saw the 'becoming' of a bilateral monopoly between government and the medical profession, in which the OMA would defend the interests of all medical doctors (specialists and GPs). In terms of reform, the government secured a deal with medical doctors that enabled it to receive federal money to cover healthcare costs.

Consolidating Ontario Medicare: managing the turbulence, 1970–90

The influence of context: drivers and shapers of medical politics

These two decades were influenced by conservative political leadership and shaped by early experience of the new deal that linked medical doctors and government together within a PFHS. This period represented a kind of golden age for medical doctors, where their commitment to the PFHS brought them significant economic gains. The exodus of medical doctors after the introduction of Medicare was not as large as anticipated (O'Donnell, 1979). However, this period would also feature increasing economic constraints as the higher cost of medical compensation in the 1970s, coupled with a global recession, triggered a period of rationalisation in healthcare. It was also marked by persistent preoccupations with satisfying the federal government's specific criteria in order to qualify for transfers. Ultimately, both medical doctors and the Ontario government were under considerable pressure to reach agreement on contentious matters.

Strategies used to accommodate and deal with the evolving context

The government introduced the Health Insurance Organisation Act in 1971, which cast a shadow over its brief honeymoon with organised medicine. The Act aimed to increase government's power to control and audit medical compensation, and prevent extra billing to patients. This was a significant policy moment, where the OMA realised that they had to get better equipped to resist government intrusion in medical affairs. The nascent OHIP of 1972, the Act respecting the Ministry of Health (1972) and the Health Disciplines Act (1974), confirmed the government's determination to develop greater capacity to intervene in medical affairs and to act as a main regulator. They also opened up the possibility of alternatives to FFS payment mechanisms for medical doctors. Proposals to redesign GP practices to serve as community health centres were discussed and promoted in early 1970s; however, the medical profession's capacity for resistance would sidetrack many progressive policy options promoted by government.

In 1978, during a period of rationalisation, the government transferred development of the fee schedule from the OMA to the Ministry of Health and imposed a significant reduction in medical compensation. This infuriated medical doctors, and a large number opted out of the public plan in response (Weiers, 1979). The government had underestimated the profession's determination to maintain control over their practice and compensation. The federal government threatened to withhold funding due to the prevalence of opting out and extra billing in Ontario, even as the federal Health Minister reminded Ontario that medical doctors needed a 'good deal' (Henderich, 1979). The Ontario government restarted negotiations with the medical profession in 1979 in the hope of restoring a more collaborative tone. In the end, medical doctors obtained an increase in compensation (11.5 per cent) and the government resisted legally prohibiting the right to opt out.

In the early 1980s, a new Minister of Health focused on reorganising primary care through models such as CHCs and HSOs, but faced resistance from the OMA, which saw them as a step toward state-controlled medicine. As a result, new models remained marginal in the system (Birch et al, 2001; Aggarwal, 2009: 121). The number of medical doctors in the province almost doubled between the 1960s and the 1980s, contributing to a startling increase in the cost of medical compensation. In negotiations with government, the OMA obtained a 30 per cent increase in compensation, using inter-provincial comparison to support their claim. The OMA argued that by ensuring appropriate compensation, it prevented an exodus of doctors and thus upheld the level of care.

When the federal government adopted the CHA, which prohibits extra billing, the OMA launched a constitutional legal challenge (CMA, 1984), and struck an alliance with far-right politicians of the moment. The Ontario election of 1985 brought a coalitional government (NDP and Liberal) to power that promised to eradicate extra billing. The OMA considered that the government was trying to erode recent gains and maintained their opposition. The federal government imposed a deadline for provinces to implement the CHA and withheld $50 million in transfer payments to Ontario. Medical doctors rallied behind the OMA's call for resistance, participating in a campaign of pressure tactics, including a legal challenge against Ontario's Health Care Accessibility Act (Bill 94, SO, 1986, c. 20) (Harrington, 1985a; Newbery, 1986), and, in 1986, staged the longest medical doctors' strike in Canadian history (25 days) (J. Ferguson, 1986).

Public opinion in Ontario was generally not supportive of the OMA and medical doctors' position, seeing their resistance to the CHA as working against people's wellbeing. The formation of the MRG, which supported the ban on extra billing, also revealed fragmentation in medical politics. The law prohibiting extra billing was adopted in July 1986 as a result of a set of convergent forces that defeated medical resistance. The Act included additional measures, including one that officially recognised the OMA as the sole body representing medical doctors. However, negotiations between the OMA and the government around compensation in 1987 ended with the government imposing a settlement. The final noteworthy event of the 1980s was passage of the Act respecting independent health facilities (Bill 147, 1989/SO, 1989, c. 59) that gave the government, through the CPSO, power to intervene in the inspection and accreditation of independent health facilities that were spreading across the province. The OMA saw this as another sign of growing bureaucratic control over medical practice in Ontario.

In the early 1990s, there were signs of change in the OMA's strategy; it published the paper *Toward a Partnership in the 1990s* and withdrew its court action against the CHA. In 1991, a sense of collaborative policy-making between the government and the OMA was tangible with the introduction of the Ontario Medical Association Dues Act (Bill 135, SO, 1991, c. 51); it created a joint committee composed of high-ranking officials from the OMA and the Ministry, giving the medical profession a voice in the future of the Ontario healthcare system.

Impact on medical politics and healthcare reforms

This second period was characterised by the government asserting itself as a main player within the healthcare system and, consequently, as a legitimate interlocutor for the medical profession. It saw a maturation of medical politics, where the OMA became more aware of the need to develop the machinery to negotiate with and oppose government when required. Medical doctors realised that, while they could voice opposition, the government could use its power to pass laws and impose its views. The medical profession achieved most of its objectives and was able to rally members of the profession in major contestations. The profession also learned that *open tent* medical politics entail risks, such as misalignment with population expectations. This period ended with a sense of policy learning, where both protagonists agreed on the benefits of a more collaborative approach. In terms of healthcare reforms, government was unable to fulfil a more ambitious reformative agenda regarding primary care. The development of alternate models of healthcare organisation and medical compensation was slowed and diluted by OMA resistance. In most negotiations during this period, the government ended up conceding to increases in compensation, a common way to buy provisional peace with medical doctors.

Recession hits: restructuring through the Social Contract and the 'Common Sense Revolution', 1990–95

The influence of context: drivers and shapers of medical politics

The relative collaboration between medical doctors and government was disrupted in 1991 as the province entered its worst recession since the early 1980s. Growing preoccupation with the cost of healthcare and the sustainability of the public system led the government to introduce the Expenditure Control Plan Statute Law Amendment Act 1993 with the objective of reducing healthcare expenses by $1 billion (Priest, 1992). Given the general hardship imposed by recession, the public and government were largely unsympathetic to doctors' complaints about their fees (Priest, 1993a). These factors set the tone for relations between the medical profession and government in this period. In 1995, the PC was back in power and promoted a 'Common Sense Revolution' that aimed to improve the province's public finances. Their political programme included creating the HSRC to rationalise the healthcare system.

Strategies used to accommodate and deal with the evolving context

In 1993, the government used coercive measures with doctors by introducing the Interim Agreement of Economic Arrangements,[39] imposing a 'hard cap'[40] on the total funding envelope for Ontario doctors, cutting the envelope by 5.5 per cent and seeking another $20 million in savings by delisting certain procedures and limiting coverage of others. It also barred medical doctors from outside Ontario from practising in the province for three years. When total billings by medical doctors exceeded the cap before the end of the year, the progressive OMA Board recommended that OHIP hold back 4.8 per cent of payments to medical doctors (CMA, 1993). There appeared to be some dissent within the OMA (and more broadly among doctors) about their duty to help reduce costs without jeopardising patient care. The OMA Council voted that doctors take nine days off per year for three years to cover the difference, a tactic that was not condoned by the OMA Board (Priest, 1993d). The Council also suggested that doctors discourage patients from consulting them for minor problems. In the years to 1996, the medical profession absorbed most of the financial constraints imposed by government. The government introduced Bill 26, the Savings and Restructuring Act, which would rescind the OMA's status as sole representative of the medical profession and increase the Minister's power over healthcare organisations and private healthcare facilities.

The OMA responded to Bill 26 and the government programme of rationalisation and restructuring with public campaigns (*Medical Post*, 1996b) that criticised the PC government's approach to fixing healthcare. OMA President Dr Bill Orovan argued that the OMA's status was essential to protecting the livelihoods of doctors, especially as funding for APPs – such as capitation models in primary care – would henceforth come from the general FFS envelope (*Medical Post*, 1996c: 22–3). On 29 January 1996, the omnibus Bill 26 was adopted, giving the government new powers to set medical doctors' fees, determine what services were medically necessary, access information in patient charts, and determine where physicians could practice (*Medical Post*, 1996c). Responding to OMA objections, the government amended the bill to include a time limit on the extraordinary powers it needed to undertake hospital restructuring.[41] This period of tension again culminated in greater openness from the OMA to engage in joint policy-making, including the development of alternative models for primary care.

Impact on medical politics and healthcare reforms

In this brief period, the government asserted its capacity to confront the medical profession and the OMA out of economic necessity. The medical profession and the OMA had to find a way of collaborating with government and of showing some understanding for its imperatives. Events in this period also demonstrated that the medical profession could move beyond voicing opposition and actually participate in solutions. During these years, the government was able to implement most of its policy agenda, at least when it came to containing the cost of medical compensation.

Primary care reform, 1996–2003

The influence of context: drivers and shapers of medical politics

The government entered this period determined to make changes. Conservative leadership sought to act rapidly and decisively to balance public finances and better manage key sectors such as healthcare. This period saw major cutbacks in public spending by the federal government that impacted on healthcare transfers to the provinces. The importance and urgency of primary care reform to address healthcare challenges was stressed during this period. Dr Duncan Sinclair, who chaired the HSRC for the government of Ontario, underlined that: 'We believe that the successful reform of the health service … will depend absolutely on the development of primary care organisations and integrated health systems.' He urged the government to act rapidly (Muncin, 1997).

Strategies used by the protagonists to accommodate and deal with the evolving context

Demonstrating its intent to collaborate with government, in 1996 the OMA's Primary Care Reform Physician Advisory Group, supported by the Ministry of Health, presented a discussion paper entitled *Primary Care Reform: A Strategy for Stability*, looking at alternative payment models for family practice. It promoted a model for GPs based on patient rostering and modified FFS. The OMA saw the proposal as an 'antidote' to Bill 26 that sought to restrict where doctors could practice by limiting billing numbers. The OMA endorsed the discussion paper and the creation of Primary Care Groups. A faction of the medical profession with a distaste for managed care opposed primary care reform on the grounds that it threatened medical doctors' autonomy and freedom of choice in practice model. Implementation of the new model was slow and incremental, with pilot projects announced only in December 1997 despite strong support from both GP and specialist OMA members (Borsellino, 1998b). The Coalition of Family Physicians of Ontario, created in 1996, stepped up efforts to gain strength within the OMA and participate in the primary care reform debate (*Medical Post*, 33(28), 19 August 1997). It also campaigned to see the OMA stripped of its role as the profession's exclusive bargaining agent, which had been granted in 1991, threatened during 1996 negotiations, and reinstated in the final 1997 Agreement. In February 1998, the government passed the Expanded Nursing Services for Patients Act (Bill 127, 1997/SO, 1997, c. 9) to 'expand the scope of practice of registered nurses who hold such a certificate by allowing them to perform certain controlled acts' (Bill 127, 1997, Explanatory Note). The OMA was involved in consultations and, barring a few minor concerns, approved of the legislation (Wansbrough, 1998).

Impact on medical politics and healthcare reforms

Overall, relations between the government and the OMA in this period were collaborative and they mutually supported a policy alternative for primary care services. The OMA played an active role in designing and promoting the model. In terms of healthcare reforms, the approach to implementing new primary care models was incremental at best. The HSRC considered it too slow and piecemeal a change, while the OMA stressed the importance of launching the reform on a solid foundation. Legislation granting NPs greater autonomy was a win for healthcare reformers who sought to increase the role of professionals other than medical doctors in primary care. The relative calm in medical politics continued into the 2000s until major dysfunctions in healthcare delivery became more salient.

A quality and accountability reformative agenda, 2003–09

The influence of context: drivers and shapers of medical politics

The election of a Liberal government in 2003 brought the promise of reinvestment in healthcare in Ontario. In addition, federal government surpluses in the early 2000s encouraged it to increase transfers to the provinces to address priorities such as reducing wait times. In 2003, Ontario introduced Bill 8, the Commitment to the Future of Medicare Act, which aligned with views expressed in the federal Romanow Commission report (2001–02). Bill 8 aimed to combat two-tier healthcare and strengthen accountability within the public healthcare system. It was a time of growing preoccupation with the quality and accessibility of care, and especially of cancer care services, for Ontario patients.

Strategies used by the protagonists to accommodate and deal with the evolving context

In Bill 8, the Liberal government promoted a series of measures that aimed to make medical doctors more accountable for their practice in hospitals and prohibit them from opting out of the public system. Negotiations with the OMA led to many amendments, including the exemption of medical doctors from accountability provisions. The government was determined to improve the quality achieved for the dollars spent in healthcare. As stated by Health Minister Smitherman: 'Together, with our wait times strategy and the emerging Ontario Health Quality Council, we will be well-positioned to achieve the best possible healthcare results for Ontarians' (quoted in Hodges, 2005). The government assembled a Health Results Team to, among other things, ensure that hospital specialists implement systems to track and reduce wait times. This represented a harder than usual policy line with medical doctors.

Meanwhile, in 2004 the OMA embarked on a long (nine-month) round of negotiations with government. Key discussions were around new mechanisms to compensate GPs in the context of primary care reform, and indexation of medical compensation. While the negotiated agreement received full support from the OMA negotiating team, the OMA Council demanded a members' vote and the strength of certain coalitions of medical specialists and GPs, opposed to any threat to their autonomy, led to the proposed deal being rejected. Specialists considered that medical doctors were being treated like government employees. The Minister amended certain sections of the agreement and contemplated imposing it unilaterally. The CMA entered the fray, seeing the government's intention as a potential breach of the CHA's requirement for binding arbitration between medical doctors and government. Finally, the government made many concessions and, in April 2005, an agreement was reached with the OMA.

At the same time, an audit process put in place by government to verify the billing practices of medical doctors was decried as an intrusion into medical practice. An inquiry was conducted and its report (Cory, 2005) was highly critical of the original medical audit system (as was the OMA), proposing 118 recommendations to improve the regulatory system. Many were implemented in a 2006 omnibus bill (Bill 171, 2006/SO, 2007, c. 10). Medical doctors were able, during this period, to largely contain the bureaucratic rationalisation of medicine. Bill 171 also formalised bilateral entities for joint policy-making between the OMA and the government around medical compensation and fee schedules.

In 2009, the Minister introduced the Regulated Health Professions Statute Law Amendment Act (Bill 179, 2009/SO, 2009, c. 26), which aimed to improve the accessibility and quality of care by authorising non-medical health professionals to perform certain regulated acts independently from medical doctors. The OMA ran newspaper ads warning Ontarians of the danger this posed, while others, including the Ontario Hospital Association, considered that medical doctors were simply trying to protect their 'turf'. (Rachlis, 2009) The CPSO saw the bill as an attempt by government to increase its control over healthcare, and criticised the inadequacy of mechanisms to support changes in professional practice. The government resisted these critiques, and adopted Bill 179.

Impact on medical politics and health reforms

Overall, this period was a complex mix of collaborative joint policy meetings between the OMA, medical doctors and the government, and conflict around medical compensation and the preservation of professional autonomy. Both medical doctors and the government were able, at key moments, to pursue their policy agendas. Operating through the OMA, medical doctors prevented the intrusion of bureaucratic rationalisers into their practice. The government resisted pressure from the OMA and introduced changes to improve access to care and gain efficiency in the utilisation of resources. The government was also successful in promoting the role of medical doctors as leaders in health policy in order to support a quality and accountability agenda.

The quality and accountability agenda: a patient-oriented project, 2010–19

The influence of context: drivers and shapers of medical politics

After the 2008 financial crisis, Ontario's economy was in recovery mode. The Conservative government in place at federal level (2006–15) targeted healthcare as a major area for policy change and sought to impose a reduction in federal health transfers (a policy that was also pursued by the Liberal government elected in 2015). In Ontario, the Drummond Report (Drummond, 2012) on deficit reduction recommended a major rationalisation of public finances. This presaged a period of difficult relations between government and the medical profession.

Strategies used by the protagonists to accommodate and deal with the evolving context

In 2010, the Liberal government of Ontario introduced the Excellent Care for All Act (Bill 46, 2010/SO, 2010, c. 14), in which new accountability measures did not apply to individual medical doctors or primary care practices. The OMA was supportive of increased accountability for boards and administrators, and of the focus on patient experience, but insisted on keeping quality evaluation in the hands of clinical leaders (Standing Committee on Justice Policy, 20 May 2010).

This period also saw hospitals and community care and mental health providers come together to propose ways to increase system efficiency. These included amending the Public Hospitals Act and redrawing the system of doctors' hospital privileges to introduce a contract model with performance requirements (Borsellino, 2010a). Medical doctors opposed the proposal, which they felt threatened their autonomous status within these organisations.

In 2011, the OMA prepared to negotiate compensation in a context where government was calling for a freeze on public service-related contracts. The government's determination was embodied in the 'white binder' – handed to the OMA at the start of negotiations – that contrasted the province's fiscal position with increases medical doctors had benefited from in recent years (Leslie, 2013a). The government demanded $1 billion in cuts to fees and programmes over four years. Minister Matthews said: 'I will not look Ontario patients in the eye and tell them they're going to have to make do with less home care and community care because we're going to have to put that money into the pockets of doctors, who are already earning an average of $362,000 a year' (quoted in Koul, 2012). When it threatened to take the unprecedented move of imposing unilateral cuts on doctors' fees, the government attracted the ire of the CMA along with the OMA and was reminded of its duty under the CHA to negotiate responsibly with medical doctors. That brought the Minister back to the table with a proposal for modest across-the-board fee cuts that proved acceptable to the OMA. The agreement included establishment of a conciliation process that promised to smooth future negotiations (Belluz, 2012b; Stuffco, 2013; Leslie, 2015b).

Midway through this arduous negotiation, medical doctors also grew concerned, after the government released *Ontario's Action Plan for Health Care* in January 2012, about what role regional health bodies, the LHINs, would have in medical compensation. The OMA assured them that physician funding would remain with the Ministry (Belluz, 2012c).

Some members of the medical profession saw this period as a game changer. For a former OMA district board director, it was a reality check: the OMA never really had representation rights: 'now the charade is over, and doctors in Ontario are beginning to realise just what a house of cards their financial future was built upon' (Goodwin, 2012). Another set of negotiations began in March 2014 with the government again insisting on cuts. Despite the interventions of a facilitator and conciliator, in January 2015, the OMA Board formally rejected the government's offer and the Minister unilaterally imposed a 2.65 per cent cut to all FFS physician payments (Leslie, 2015a). The OMA filed a Canadian Charter challenge against the Government of Ontario that aimed to introduce binding arbitration mechanisms into the negotiation process.[42] The government was concerned that arbitrator decisions failed to consider a province's fiscal reality (Leslie, 2016).

In response to the government's actions, a group calling themselves Concerned Ontario Doctors came to life in the fall of 2015, and launched a media campaign and rally against funding cuts. The emergence of this group of doctors on the right of the political spectrum changed the nature of medical politics in the province.

When the government and the OMA Council arrived with a proposed Physician Services Agreement in 2016, some felt that it presented an opportunity to restore collaboration. OMA President Dr Virginia Walley recommended approving the agreement and working out the finer points later.

At the same time, the government was looking for ways to better integrate primary care into the healthcare system. The Strengthening Primary Care Expert Advisory Committee (Price-Baker Commission) (2015) proposed decentralising funding and creating 'Patient Care Groups' as local organisations with broad care mandates (Marchildon and Hutchison, 2016, note 736). The OMA opposed this form of funding as it would undermine its right to represent medical doctors and negotiate on their behalf directly with government (Marchildon and Hutchison, 2016, note 737). Monopoly representation by the OMA was at stake with the legislation, the Patients First Act, proposed around these local organisations.

The OMA continued efforts to gain support for the Physician Services Agreement, which, importantly, withdrew sections of the Patients First Act that would have given LHINs significant oversight over medical doctors. The deal also allowed the OMA to continue its court fight for binding arbitration. A broad coalition supported the agreement, illustrating that medical politics was, momentarily at least, embedded in the province's broader health policy momentum. The defeat, in a members' vote, of the Agreement (Boyle, 2016a, 2017a) testified to the consolidation of opposing factions in medical politics. The Coalition, including DoctorsOntario and Concerned Ontario Doctors, campaigned hard against the agreement and more globally against the OMA's monopoly over representation of medical doctors.[43]

In 2017, Minister Hoskins outlined implications of the OMA being recognised as a public sector union as part of the Agreement: doctors' earnings would be made public and they would no longer be able to incorporate individually (Boyle, 2016b). These were high cost for stabilising their political machine. The Coalition continued to oppose the Agreement (Boyle, 2016a) while hundreds of other doctors urged the OMA and the Ministry to return to the table and supported the OMA as the unified voice of the profession (Bronca, 2016a). The Coalition of Ontario Doctors staged what some called a 'coup' to overthrow the OMA's executive, underscoring that medical politics was far from being a unified front in Ontario (Boyle, 2017b).

As the province headed into elections in 2018, the OMA and Concerned Ontario Doctors each produced ad campaign with different messages. Elections on 7 June 2018 saw the end of 15 years of Liberal government and the election of the PCs under Premier Doug Ford. Ontario's medical doctors, without an agreement on fees since 2014, signed a deal that was considered a sensible compromise in February 2019.

Ultimately, this period was one of confrontation. Protagonists entered the mediated space with clear diverging positions, and fought with all the means at their disposal to come out on top. The government relied on the legislature to impose its views on medical doctors, and medical doctors did not hesitate to use the courts along with various other strategies to uphold their positions.

Impacts on medical politics and health reforms

In the years up to the election of the PC in 2018, the government was able to impose a reduction in the cost of medical compensation and demonstrated its ability to stand up to the medical association and withstand its resistance. The government's willingness to enter into overt conflict with the medical profession around compensation had a major impact on the configuration of medical politics in Ontario. It led to the emergence of various factions within the profession – signs of pluralism in medical politics – and the ascendance of right-wing medical politics. It also saw the emergence of more progressive medical doctors who tried to oppose the views of conservative factions and collaborate with government. Monopoly representation by the OMA was contested. The CMA also appeared as a political force to counter any weakening of the bargaining power of medical doctors. The focus on binding arbitration was emblematic of their concerns.

While the government was able to play hardball on medical compensation, its ability to bring about significant change in the relation between the medical profession and the PFHS was less clear. Changing the social compact between medical doctors and the system through the implementation of new accountability mechanisms and a more decentralised approach to the management of medical affairs appeared much more difficult than imposing reductions in medical compensation. In the end, medical politics became more polarised during this period, but the way medical doctors operate within the health system remained more or less the same. In addition, this period revealed medical politics as an institution in becoming where the legitimacy of the OMA as the main vehicle to defend medical aspirations and interests could still be contested.

Notes

[1] Canada Health Act, R.S.C., 1985, c. C-6. See: https://laws-lois.justice.gc.ca/eng/acts/c-6/fulltext.html

[2] See: https://laws-lois.justice.gc.ca/eng/acts/c-6/fulltext.html

[3] Rochon, J. (Commission d'enquête sur les services de santé et les services sociaux) (1988) Rapport de la Commission d'enquête sur les services de santé et les services sociaux. Québec: Publications du Québec, p 221.

[4] In 2014, the average proportion of Canadians without a family doctor was 14.9 per cent, while in Québec it was 25.2 per cent. See www150.statcan.gc.ca/n1/pub/82-625-x/2015001/article/14177-eng.htm

[5] https://plus.lapresse.ca/screens/f54e8b5f-050e-442e-91f1-f2d0fcf71a8a__7C___0.html

[6] 'MDs' pamphlets in waiting rooms aimed at OMSIP', 2 August 1966.

[7] 'Doctors raised fees 15 per cent, Dymond says in noting OMSIP rise'.

[8] www.historymuseum.ca/cmc/exhibitions/hist/medicare/medic-6h02e.shtml

[9] 'With the advent of government sponsored health insurance physician control over provincial and federal health organizations declined. Physicians were replaced in positions of authority by health bureaucrats, planners, managers and accountants. This was true at all levels. In Ontario, for example, all health ministers until 1968 had been physicians, after that time (apart from a brief period [the Dr Potter's ministry]) all health ministers have been laypersons' (Coburn, 1993: 132).

[10] SO, 1975, c. 47, ss. 3(2).

[11] SO, 1986, c. 20, ss. 3(2)a.

[12] Comparing strikes that occurred in Winnipeg (1933–34), Saskatchewan (1962) and Québec (1970).

[13] www.ola.org/en/legislative-business/committees/social-development/parliament-35/transcript/committee-transcript-1991-aug-06

[14] www.ola.org/en/legislative-business/committees/social-development/parliament-35/transcript/committee-transcript-1991-aug-26#P459_160163

[15] www.ola.org/en/legislative-business/committees/social-development/parliament-35/transcript/committee-transcript-1991-aug-28#P90_20669

[16] *Ontario Hansard*, 5 November 1991, Hon Ms Lankin, http://hansardindex.ontla.on.ca/hansardetitle/35-1/l080-75.html

[17] SO, 1991, c. 51, s. 2.

[18] SO, 1991, c. 51, ss. 3(1). Paragraph 5(1) provides that if a physician does not pay his [sic] dues, the general manager of the OHIP can deduct the required amount and pay it to the OMA.

[19] www.ola.org/en/legislative-business/committees/social-development/parliament-35/transcript/committee-transcript-1991-dec-02

[20] SO, 1993, c. 32, ss. 1(1) and 1(2).

[21] SO, 1993, c. 32, ss. 1(1) and 1(2), 23.

[22] 'The OMA recognizes the need for significant restructuring within hospitals and it supports the general thrust of this aspect of Bill 26. However, the OMA believes these

powers should be viewed as extraordinary and must be time limited. Recently proposed amendments to Bill 26 from the government indicate that the government is following the OMA's advice in this matter' (https://www.ola.org/en/legislative-business/committees/general-government/parliament-36/transcripts/committee-transcript-1996-jan-19).

23 www.ola.org/en/legislative-business/committees/justice-social-policy/parliament-38/transcripts/committee-transcript-2004-feb-26.

24 SO, 2004, c. 13, s. 2, enacting ss. 7(2) and (4) to the Ministry of Health Appeal and Review Board Act 1998.

25 SO, 2004, c. 13, s. 10: 'There can be no doubt that the present audit system has had a debilitating – and, in some cases, devastating – effect on the physicians of Ontario, their families, their practices and their patients, and as well a negative impact on the delivery of health services in the Province.'

26 SO, 2004, c. 13, ss. 2(1), enacting s. 5.1(1) of the Health Insurance Act.

27 SO, 2004, c. 13, ss. 2(1), enacting s. 5.1(5) of the Health Insurance Act.

28 www.ola.org/en/legislative-business/committees/social-policy/parliament-39/transcripts/committee-transcript-2009-sep-29

29 Subsection 24.1(2) of Bill 179, 2009, that added Section 5.0.1 to the Regulated Health Professions Act 1991. It is in the law as adopted: SO, 2009, c. 26, ss. 24.1(2).

30 www.ctvnews.ca/health/ontario-doctors-crying-foul-over-upcoming-fee-cut-1.2578338

31 Ontario Legislative Assembly, Dr Stephen Chris, 13 November 2016: https://www.ola.org/en/legislative-business/committees/legislative-assembly/parliament-41/transcripts/committee-transcript-2016-nov-14#P246_52171

32 Formerly the Coalition of Family Physicians and Specialists of Ontario. It was created in 1996 and changed its name to 'DoctorsOntario' in 2013. Ontario Legislative Assembly, Dr Stephen Chris, 13 November 2016: www.ola.org/en/legislative-business/committees/legislative-assembly/parliament-41/transcripts/committee-transcript-2016-nov-14

33 https://www.ola.org/en/legislative-business/committees/legislative-assembly/parliament-41/transcripts/committee-transcript-2016-nov-21

34 Ontario Legislative Assembly, 23 November 2016: www.ola.org/en/legislative-business/committees/legislative-assembly/parliament-41/transcripts/committee-transcript-2016-nov-23

35 http://www.carenotcuts.ca/

36 https://www.newswire.ca/news-releases/oma-brings-awareness-to-wait-times-crisis-in-new-campaign-677290843.html

37 https://www.oma.org/newsroom/news/2018/mar/oma-brings-awareness-to-wait-times-crisis-in-new-campaign/

38 www.carenotcuts.ca

39 Tom Dickson, OMA President, opening comments.

40 Tom Dickson, OMA President, opening comments.

41 'The OMA recognizes the need for significant restructuring within hospitals and it supports the general thrust of this aspect of Bill 26. However, the OMA believes these powers should be viewed as extraordinary and must be time limited. Recently proposed amendments to Bill 26 from the government indicate that the government is following the OMA's advice in this matter': www.ola.org/en/legislative-business/committees/general-government/parliament-36/transcripts/committee-transcript-1996-jan-19#P255_63752

42 www.oma.org/newsroom/news/2015/oct/to-help-protect-patient-focused-care-ontarios-doctors-file-charter-challenge-against-ontario-government/

43 http://www.carenotcuts.ca/

The role of medical doctors in healthcare reforms in the NHS in England

For a better understanding of the historical role played by medical doctors in the NHS healthcare reforms, we need a few preliminary words on the process of law-making to reform the healthcare system in England.

Usually, the reformative process is ignited by an inquiry or policy proposal. In the early years of the NHS, the government established Royal Commissions as ad hoc committees (House of Lords, 2007) tasked to lead investigations that triggered reforms. This long and burdensome process later gave way to more targeted inquiries to inform policy changes (for example, the Griffiths Report or NHS Management Inquiry, 1983).

The government could also put forward reform strategies and policy proposals in a publicly released White Paper, offering stakeholders the opportunity to provide written or oral responses that are valuable in highlighting any controversial areas. Parliament has, at times, been convened to debate responses to White Papers before the government proceeds with a formal legislative proposal or Bill to be 'read' (examined and debated) three times in Parliament (Select Committee on the Constitution, 2017–19). The draft law is then presented either to the House of Commons or the House of Lords (or sometimes both) and, if passed, receives Royal Assent before becoming law.

While stakeholders are not invited to interact directly in the House of Lords or the House of Commons, their support or objections are relayed by Lords or members of the House of Commons who act as unofficial spokespersons because their political interests align or because they are themselves members of a Royal College of Medicine or the British Medical Association (BMA) (Select committee on the Constitution, 2017: 14). The Second Reading of a Bill provides a forum for these exchanges, and the written reports are revelatory of the positions held by government and the medical profession on proposed healthcare reforms (Germain, 2019).

Part 1: Case history

Creating the NHS, pre-1948

In 1944, as the Second World War still raged, plans for the National Health Service were set out in a White Paper. The political agenda in the UK in the immediate post-war period was driven by ambitions to change healthcare provision. The plan centred on two principles: the creation of a comprehensive healthcare service and the guarantee of free access to care for all citizens. Enshrined in law in 1946, the policy framework did not, however, address the fragmentation of healthcare services and the existence of charges for hospital care (Webster, 1988).

The plan was not the first effort to remodel healthcare services. In June 1942, the BMA approved, by a small majority, a policy design for a healthcare system based on universal access (Honigsbaum, 1989) that built on the existing National Health Insurance (NHI) scheme (Ham, 2009). This would have allowed medical professionals to maintain their independent status. GPs were particularly concerned with the potential expanded role, in the 1944 White Paper, of municipal authorities, which could encroach on their autonomy and clinical freedom.

The government was toying with the idea of turning GPs into salaried, municipally controlled workers. Some would work in local health centres overseen by local authorities; others would keep operating in single practices on the basis of contractual arrangements with a central medical board and would be free to also take on private patients (Ministry of Health and Department of Health for Scotland, 1944: v). A 'contractual relationship' between the GP and the 'public authority' was considered necessary to guarantee that 'the services which the people [were receiving were] the services which they need[ed] (and for which they [were to] be paying in taxation or otherwise)' (Ministry of Health and Department of Health for Scotland, 1944: v).

The White Paper emphasised government's willingness to enter into a dialogue with the medical profession as '[it] want[ed] [its] proposals to be freely examined and discussed' and to have 'constructive criticism of them, in the hope that the legislative proposals ... may follow quickly' (Ministry of Health and Department of Health for Scotland, 1944: Introductory). Despite the government's expression of good will, the BMA maintained its opposition to free-for-all universalism and preference for extending the NHI (Pater, 1981).

The end of the war coincided with Labour winning its first general election and the 'audacious' appointment of Aneurin Bevan as Minister for Health and Housing (Webster, 1988). Bevan was in favour of the nationalisation of charitable and municipal hospitals to address issues of financing and equitable distribution of services. Hospital nationalisation was perceived as a means to give specialist medical doctors 'what they wanted as well as what Bevan wanted' (Glennerster, 1995: 51). Lord Moran, President of the Royal College of Physicians at the time, explicitly suggested that doctors would have accepted to enter the NHS if the control of hospitals had been removed from municipal authorities (Titmuss, 1958).

The medical profession was on board with the principle of a national health service, but did not agree with all aspects of the plan as imagined by Bevan.

Throughout the ensuing negotiations, the medical profession repeatedly tested the limits of what they could demand as a way of highlighting potential sticking points, but maintained steadfast opposition to the idea of GPs becoming public servants (Klein, 2013).

To avoid open conflict, Bevan decided to put his final proposal before Parliament without giving the whole of the medical profession an opportunity to scrutinise the plan (Eckstein, 1958; Rintala, 2003). Only in the final round of discussions did Bevan open the floor to input from medical doctors. This tactic was not well received by the BMA and made subsequent exchanges more complex (Greener, 2009). The medical profession's grievances were, however, relayed by their union during the second reading of the foundational Bill in the House of Commons in April 1946.

The antagonistic relationship between the government and the profession contrasted with the collaborative tone adopted by the government in the 1944 White Paper. In some instances, medical doctors' profound discontent with the prospect of losing professional autonomy was communicated through Members of Parliament (MPs). Bevan, however, stood firm and rebutted 'the doctors' [claim] that the proposals of the Bill amount[ed] to direction' because he strongly believed that 'there [was] no direction involved at all' (House of Commons, 1946: col 54).

Most vocal in representing the medical profession's perspective was a Conservative MP, Richard Law, who, directly addressing Bevan in the Commons, stated that 'The British Hospital Association and the British Medical Association [were] opposed to this Bill' and added that '[t]he British Dental Association [was] also opposed to this Bill, and [that] the three Royal Colleges [had] criticized it with varying emphasis' (House of Commons, 1946: col 64). He went as far as affirming that 'the plain fact [was] that everybody of informed and expert opinion outside [the] House [was] against the Minister on one part of the Bill or another' (House of Commons, 1946: col 66).

In reality, Bevan had engaged in conversations on the main principles of the plan with select leaders of the medical profession (Rintala, 2003). He favoured dealing with hospital specialists because the Royal Colleges (representing specialists) could make decisions without prior consultation of their members. Conversely, the BMA, mainly representing GPs, operated through full consultation and member votes (Honigsbaum, 1989).

Bevan attempted to divide the medical profession (Ham, 2009), and partially succeeded, luring on board the Royal Colleges to stave off BMA opposition (Klein, 2013). Specialists were promised flexible working conditions, special status in teaching hospitals and the possibility of practising privately in NHS hospitals. In his own words, Bevan had 'stuffed their mouths with gold' (quoted in Abel-Smith, 1964: 480). On the contrary, only minimal concessions were made to GPs, and they remained fearful of losing their status as independent contractors right up until publication of the NHS Act 1946.

Charles Hill, one of the most vocal GP spokespeople, explicitly called on citizens to make sure 'that [their] doctor d[id] not become the state's doctor' (quoted in Rivett, 1998: 36). Further GP concerns related to being forced to work in less affluent parts of the country and losing the right to be paid a goodwill when selling practices. Eventually, the GPs' dogged resistance forced Bevan to make more substantial concessions, including the promise that their autonomy and freedom would not be compromised (Pater, 1981).

Despite these concessions, in January 1948 GPs still voted almost unanimously (84 per cent) against the proposed format of the NHS in a plebiscite organised by the BMA (Morrell, 1998). Bevan rejected the medical profession's counterproposal of a service that did not cover the totality of the population. He was also keen to eliminate insurance contributions (Ham, 2009). He did, however, accept that GPs would be paid on a capitation basis, renouncing his intention to institute a salaried service.

As a part of the 'concordat' (Klein, 2013), the State committed to use caution when interfering in medical training and internal politics. The medical profession had rejected earlier proposals for the State to take control of medical education. A few months later, the BMA recommended that its members accept the NHS plan, but many GPs retained a sense of unease and contempt (Rivett, 1998). In the final plebiscite, 54 per cent voted against discussions with the Minister (and 66 per cent opposed further negotiations), but the plan was eventually approved.

Thirty years of 'consensus': the NHS between 1948 and 1979

Following the open debates and confrontations that occupied the first half of 1948, Bevan subsequently privileged discreet negotiations between civil servants and representatives of the medical profession as a way of incorporating interest groups in the decision-making process (Eckstein, 1960). Medical professionals were awarded between 30 per cent and 40 per cent of administrative positions in NHS healthcare organisations on the grounds that their expertise was needed in 'medical aspects of management' (Klein, 2013).

The government and medical doctors made concerted efforts to agree and make the system work successfully. This did not mean that what Klein (2013) called their 'double bed' relationship was entirely free from confrontation. However, at the end of the 1950s, two-thirds of the medical profession were still in favour of the NHS arrangement.

From its inception, running the NHS proved more expensive than budgeted, and much more than what Parliament expected (Ham, 2009). In 1950, a *BMJ* Editorial claimed that the service was headed towards bankruptcy

(BMJ, 1950). Demands for greater funding concentrated especially on health system infrastructure, as many Victorian-era hospital buildings had not been renovated since the 19th century (Abel and Lewin, 1959).

A senior civil servant, Sir Cyril Jones, suggested that expenditure would be brought under control only when doctors were stripped of managerial responsibilities in NHS facilities (Jones, 1950). Even Bevan considered that 'doctors had secured too great a degree of control over hospital management committees, and were pursuing a perfectionist policy without regard to the financial limits which had necessarily to be imposed on this service as on other public services' (cited in Klein, 2013: 27).

The 1950s were a decade of 'consolidation', greatly needed after the confrontations of the 1940s (Klein, 2013). The transformation of specialists into salaried hospital employees dramatically changed their relationship with GPs. GPs maintained their gatekeeper function (Dowling, 2000), but the relationship of mutual dependency that had been fundamentally demand-led (and controlled by GPs) was turned on its head. Salaried specialists decided on what terms healthcare services would be provided (Greener, 2009). The Cohen Committee (Central Health Services Committee, 1954) suggested that given that the status and prestige of GPs was equal to that of other medical specialties, their training should follow a similar path, but this suggestion was not acted on (Rivett, 1998).

The workload and duties of GPs changed substantially in the post-1948 arrangement. They faced a steep increase in the number of patients seeking healthcare services, while also having to write prescriptions and issue health certificates (Greener, 2009). Morale was generally low, especially as government resources were increasingly channelled towards hospital care. There also appeared to be a crisis of representation, as many GPs were still resentful of the BMA's lack of effectiveness during negotiations around the creation of the NHS (Greener, 2009). In 1952, the Royal College of General Practitioners (RCGP) was founded (despite the opposition of the other Royal Colleges), giving GPs a new representative body.

GPs were paid a flat capitation fee, as determined by the Spens report (Parliament, 1948). Many GPs felt that the inability to also see private patients unfairly impacted their remuneration. Low compensation led to stagnation in the recruitment of GPs in the initial years of the NHS (Godber, 1975). Pay disputes became a common theme during the 1950s, partially fuelled by the election, in 1951, of a Conservative government that was ideologically opposed to overspending. The medical profession expressed scepticism about the 'utopian finances of the Welfare State' (BMJ, 1950: 1262).

GP compensation improved in 1952 when the capitation system was replaced with a more favourable payment formula agreed in a new deal negotiated with GPs. This linked pay increases with improvements in general practice (Greener, 2009). The Report of the Royal Commission on Doctors' and Dentists' Remuneration (1960) suggested that doctors' earnings were effectively low and had fallen behind those of comparable occupations. The report recommended increasing pay levels as well as establishing a permanent review body (Klein, 2013).

In 1959, a group of BMA specialists called for a 10-year investment plan in the acute care sector (mentioned in Klein, 2013: 54). A subsequent BMA report went to the extreme of invoking a return to an insurance-based system in order to generate resources (BMA, 1969). In the following years, the government poured massive resources into the healthcare system and in particular into improving and updating hospital facilities. Under *A Hospital Plan for England and Wales* (Minister of Health, 1962), the NHS undertook substantial infrastructure investments and created District General Hospitals (DGHs).

For their part, GPs were unhappy with the fact that payments from the revised capitation formula did not take into consideration the quality of service provided for practices of comparable size. A group of GPs formed the new General Practitioners' Association to push the BMA into action (Rivett, 1998). In 1963, the BMA duly passed a motion to improve the financial status of GPs (Klein, 2013).

The most significant development in general practice in the first 20 years of the NHS (Ham, 2009) was the submission in 1965 of a Charter for the Family Doctor Service by Dr James Cameron, a prominent spokesperson and Chair of the General Medical Services Committee (GMSC). Aiming to improve working conditions, the Charter became popular among GPs and was rapidly adopted by the BMA.

Dr Cameron asked fellow GPs to pressure government during contract negotiations by signing undated resignation letters. More than 14,000 letters were accordingly sent to the BMA. After months of bargaining, the new contract was finally agreed in 1966. It included a 30 per cent increase in pay, reimbursement for ancillary staff, a contribution to the cost of practice premises, funding for postgraduate training and loans to modernise buildings (Loudon et al, 1998).

Importantly, this was the first time GPs threatened to withdraw their services altogether from the NHS. The BMA was aware of the uneasiness among GPs but struggled to effectively convey their unhappiness as it was intent on portraying itself as the unified voice for the whole medical profession (Greener, 2009). This crisis of representation was severe enough that in 1972 the BMA commissioned an external review of its constitution and organisation, undertaken by an eminent civil servant and industrialist, Sir Paul Chambers (BMJ, 1972). In taking stock of the NHS' second decade, Klein (2013) suggests that 'from being an oasis of industrial peace, the NHS became relatively dispute-prone' (2013: 51).

Pressures on public finances were mounting in the 1970s and hospitals were seen as too expensive and too large and impersonal (Turner, 1995).

Pay conditions become problematic, with high inflation requiring repeated adjustment. Doctors' compensation was falling behind relative to other professions: between 1975 and 1977 the overall pay conditions for doctors worsened by 20 per cent (Klein, 2013).

In October 1975, junior doctors in Leicester went on strike over pay, and the protest quickly spread across the country, encouraged by medical unions. This was the first time ever that the medical profession had withdrawn services, despite having threatened to do so in 1911 and 1946. The splintering of medical representation became apparent, with the BMA and the Royal Colleges – perceived to be elitist and out of date – having to compete with the more activist Medical Practitioners' Union for membership, especially around the time of the strike (Greener, 2009).

The dispute with government was eventually resolved through a bonified pay settlement and junior doctors were thereafter compensated for virtually all worked hours, including overtime (Klein, 2013). This arrangement was criticised by senior members of the profession on the grounds that it reduced the pay differential between them and the junior doctors. In their view, it turned medical professionals into industrial workers: 'technologists rather than doctors' (Fox, 1976).

Specialists had threatened to withdraw their services in 1974, something that the Royal Colleges saw as a potentially dangerous move that would erode the trust between doctors and patients (BMJ, 1975). According to the Royal Colleges and the BMA, the profession had a 'special responsibility not to create conflict purely to further the advantage of its own members' (BMJ, 1977).

Doctors reacted promptly against their representatives for what they saw as an intrusion of their domain. It led to extreme consequences such as the blacklisting of operating theatres in hospitals and the lengthening of waiting lists. The government eventually awarded specialists a 9 per cent pay increase, while the maximum expected prior to the strikes had been 5 per cent.

The newly elected Conservative government of 1971, particularly its Minister of Health Keith Josef, resurfaced the idea of giving state managers control over chronic and acute services (DHSS, 1971). Changes in the management of the healthcare systems were aimed at improving efficiency (Ham, 2009). The subsequent Conservative plan to abolish the regional tier of administration controlled by doctors met with stern opposition from the medical profession. It was one of the significant concessions made by Bevan in 1948 to gain doctors' approval for the NHS (Greener, 2009). An Editorial in the BMJ raised questions about 'the extent to which the principles of organisation and related methods should be introduced into a medical service' (BMJ, 1969: 329). The plan was radical in that political appointees would become area board members rather than individuals representing the medical profession (or local authorities).

Exchanges in Parliament regarding the reorganisation Bill were brief and did not raise many controversies, but the profession's strenuous defence of its clinical autonomy was a key feature. A Fellow of the Royal College of Surgeons, Lord Brock, explained that 'many members of the medical profession [were] concerned that administrative revision ha[d] become an end in itself and that the ability to practice good medicine [was] impaired. [Doctors were] concerned that too much control, too much supervision, too much regimentation may not only be irksome and frustrating to those in the profession, but may adversely influence future recruitment'. He added that 'in spite of assurance that clinical freedom [would] be preserved, many doctors fear[ed] that impairment of their clinical and medical freedom [would] result from a too rigid bureaucratic control, however desirable this bureaucratic control may be in the non-medical affairs of the organisation and implementation of the National Health Service' (House of Lords, 1973: 95–7).

Like previous Labour governments, the Conservatives caved in to pressure and restored doctors' decision-making roles in the regional structure of the NHS (Secretary of State for Health and Social Services, 1972). The medical profession was thus once again given a key role in the new governance arrangements (Ham, 2009) in full control of the decision-making machinery (Klein, 2013).

Following the Labour government's return to power in 1974, the new Secretary of State, Barbara Castle, wanted to send a strong signal that times were changing for the medical profession by suppressing the practice of 'paybeds'. Introduced in 1946 as part of the agreement between Bevan and specialist doctors, pay-beds enabled specialists to use NHS hospital beds for their private practice patients. Labour's election platform had promised to abolish this arrangement, and a strike was organised by medical unions across the country to force the closure of private wings (Greener, 2009).

Meanwhile, Minister of Health David Owen was engaged in contract negotiations with specialists, who were willing to accept the separation of private practice from the NHS in exchange for financial incentives, but opposed a ban on private practice (Klein, 2013). The BMA and the Hospital Consultants' and Specialists' Association intervened in support of the specialists' position, threatening service withdrawal and refusing to enter into negotiations with government.

In December 1974, specialists began a 16-week work-to-rule action (Rivett, 1998). Further proposals presented by the government in May 1975 were rejected by the BMA, the Royal Colleges, the Hospital Consultants and Specialists' Association and private insurers. Eventually, through arbitration, the right of specialists to work in both private and public practice was maintained – but separated from the NHS – and a limit was set on the use of private beds (Klein, 2013).

The Thatcher and Major era: consensual disagreement, 1979–97

The 1980s can be seen as a period of both continuity and contrast with the previous decade (Greener, 2009). There were further episodes of protest by the medical profession, but the government was far less willing to resort to corporatist policy-making. The medical profession was no longer regarded as a valued partner in policy-making, but rather as an actor-group with vested interests that were often poorly aligned with the needs of the healthcare system.

In the context of rising public accounts deficits, a priority for Prime Minister Margaret Thatcher's government was to simplify and decentralise the NHS, effectively reversing the centralisation of the 1974 reforms (Greener, 2009). Dissatisfaction was shared by the medical profession, who believed that the reforms had inserted a wedge between administrators and clinicians, compromising the partnership between those running and those working in the service (*BMJ*, 1978).

The government sought ways to rationalise services and to make more efficient use of existing resources (Ham, 2009). First, it abolished a management tier by combining existing administrative structures, creating 192 District Health Authorities (DHAs) in 1982 under the banner of localism (Klein, 2013). Medical representation was assured, with one GP and one specialist on the internal decision-making body of DHAs. Second, it shifted attention to organisational dynamics (Nairne, 1983), commissioning an external review to understand how to best manage the NHS.

Thatcher chose Roy Griffiths, deputy chair and managing director of Sainsbury's, a supermarket chain, to conduct the inquiry. Its landmark report (DHSS, 1983) opened a new chapter in the relationship between the government and the medical profession. Griffiths concluded that the NHS was not using resources efficiently and nor was it focused on patient needs (Ham, 2009).

A key issue was the absence of individuals responsible for overall decision-making and performance. Griffiths famously used the metaphor of Florence Nightingale armed with her lantern aimlessly wandering through the corridors of the NHS in an attempt to find somebody in charge (DHSS, 1983). He recommended devolving responsibilities to local managers, who would, in turn, be accountable to local people and to central government. The government was to refrain from micro-managing the NHS, and should push the NHS to become more business-like. The conservative Thatcher government enthusiastically adopted Griffiths' recommendations and introduced a whole new cadre of general managers into the NHS, along with a drive to increase accountability.

The medical profession was highly sceptical of these business ideas, which, in its view, went against good patient care as defined by professional autonomy (Day and Klein, 1985). Interestingly, Griffiths suggested that doctors were the 'natural managers' of the service and should accept that managerial responsibilities went hand in hand with clinical freedom. The BMA did not adhere to this view (Rivett, 1998). Hospital specialists in particular rebuffed Griffiths' proposals but, despite opposition, 'corporate rationalisers' (Alford, 1975) became an integral part of the NHS hierarchy, challenging the role played up to that point by the medical profession.

In an attempt to reduce overall public expenditure, a review initiated by Secretary of State Norman Foster and Minister for Health Kenneth Clarke in 1984 contemplated changes to GP services. The Thatcher government wanted to show that the State was getting value for money and sought to identify potential savings and assess whether the medical profession was generating efficiency (Greener, 2009).

Performance indicators were introduced, initially focusing on clinical activity outputs. Advances in health economics led to increased scrutiny of the medical profession. Doctors were required to employ evidence-based arguments to support their decisions and come up with ways of making more efficient use of scarce public resources (Crinson, 2009).

By the end of the decade, further reforms appeared on the government agenda. Underfunding of the service had become a dominant issue, with an accumulated shortfall of £1.8 billion between 1981/82 and 1987/88 (Robinson, 1988). Moreover, public dissatisfaction with the NHS grew from 25 per cent in 1983 to almost 50 per cent in 1989 (Judge and Solomon, 1993). Armed with a commissioned survey on hospital services showing widespread bed and staff shortages and cancelled surgeries, the BMA requested additional resources from government (Central Committee for Hospital Medical Services, 1988).

Thatcher had just won her third consecutive mandate in the 1987 General Election and wanted to use this position of power to introduce even more radical reforms. From her perspective, 'the NHS had become a pointless financial pit', with providers blaming government for all its problems (Klein, 2013: 141). Additionally, she saw the views of the Royal Colleges opposing the power of the State to impose budgetary constraints as a betrayal of the original concordat underpinning the creation of the NHS in 1948 (Klein, 2013).

Moving away from the tradition of establishing a Royal Commission to examine the situation, Thatcher took charge directly, chairing a review of the NHS. The Cabinet Committee (Timmins, 1995) she assembled was composed of civil servants and political advisers, intentionally selected because they did not represent the interests of the medical profession (Day and Klein, 1991). The BMA was explicitly excluded from participating in this review (Lee-Potter, 1997). This inevitably set up a collision course with the government based more on the review process than its substance (Day and Klein, 1992).

In the evidence it submitted to the review, the BMA, which was suffering from a dip in membership due to increased militancy and heterogeneity in the workforce (Greener, 2002), adopted a conservative stance. It argued that the NHS needed only a small adjustment in funding and that embarking on major structural reforms would be a mistake (*BMJ*, 1988).

The new Secretary of State for Health, Kenneth Clarke, took the helm of the reform programme in June 1988. Like Bevan in the 1940s, Clarke decided against consulting widely with the medical profession (Rintala, 2003). His vision centred on a radically new arrangement for the delivery of healthcare services based on a separation between purchasers and providers (Klein, 2013).

Clarke wanted to make hospitals self-governing and independent from centralised control, but also wanted to use consumer choice to drive efficiency (Klein, 2013). GP fundholders were to be given a budget to purchase care from hospitals and community healthcare providers on behalf of their patients and DHAs. Following the lead of an American health economist visiting the Nuffield Trusts, Alain Enthoven, Clarke wanted to create an internal market in the NHS where autonomous hospital providers would compete for resources.

Interestingly, the *BMJ* had previously published opinion pieces on the merits of some of Clarke's ideas, particularly around the need for incentives in the service and the view that the NHS was in a gridlock that made changes very difficult (*BMJ*, 1985). The White Paper Clarke released left the funding model untouched and concentrated on changing the dynamics driving the NHS (Klein, 2013).

At the same time, a new GP contract was being negotiated, with government keen on achieving quick agreement with the medical profession. However, the contract proposal would be repeatedly reviewed and modified over the next decade. Local committees of GPs expressed particularly strong opposition to the proposal on the table, threatening to resign from the NHS if their requests were not accommodated (General Medical Services Committee, 1989).

A tentative agreement was reached in May 1989 with concessions on both sides, but the secrecy of the negotiations left rank-and-file professionals uneasy (Klein, 2013). Eventually, GPs rejected the proposed compensation package, metaphorically suggesting that the negotiators should be hanged (General Medical Services Committee, 1990).

Unfazed, Clarke proceeded to implement the consumer-oriented changes. GPs did not believe a contract could be imposed without their consent, but were proven quite wrong. Beyond achieving a few marginal concessions, the medical profession suffered a humiliating defeat (Klein, 2013).

In January 1989, the launch of the White Paper *Working for Patients* (Secretaries of State of Health, Wales, Northern Ireland, and Scotland,

1989) received extensive media coverage. It set off 'the most serious conflict in the history [to date] of the NHS' (Klein, 2013: 140). In many ways, it represented a decisive break from the founding principles and institutional values of the NHS.

Clarke avoided consulting the medical profession on this major policy change (Greener, 2009), claiming that doctors generally 'reach(ed) for their wallets' in consultations, and that piloting the reform would have facilitated its 'sabotage' by the medical profession (quoted in Timmins, 1995). He was clearly ready for a fight: 'I told colleagues we were going into Tavistock House [the headquarters of the BMA], lifting most of the tablets of stone and smashing them on the pavement in front of their eyes' (quoted in Timmins, 1995).

The medical profession attempted to influence the course of events, both in private and in public through a well-funded campaign (Crinson, 2009), but had little impact during the consultation period or with Parliament (Grabham, 1994). Exchanges continued to be inflammatory and presaged what would unfold in negotiations around the draft legislation later that year.

The *Working for Patients* White Paper was discussed in Parliament on five occasions between February and October 1989. Unsurprisingly, MPs on both sides of the aisle had strong views about the proposal. Labour saw 'the outcome of the review [as having] a dramatic and electrifying effect on the medical profession' (House of Commons, 1989a: col 25), and stressed that government had not anticipated such strong opposition from medical organisations. Labour MPs believed '[t]he Government [had] done some terribly foolish things in relation to health. They [had] done nothing more foolish than slamming the door on the heads of the royal colleges ... [as] they [did] not consult the colleges about their plans for the future' (House of Commons, 1989a: cols 43–44).

Conversely, they praised the BMA: '[t]he thoroughness with which the doctors went about their consultations stands in marked contrast with the total failure of the Government to carry out any consultations' (House of Commons, 1989a: col 71). A joint statement put out by the Royal Colleges was read in the House of Commons explaining that '[doctors] oppose[d] medical treatment based on guess, so [they had to] regret the treatment of a whole health service on a hunch' (House of Commons, 1989a: col 26).

Clarke nonetheless stood firm and accused Labour of 'compound[ing] confusion for short-term political reasons' (House of Commons, 1989a: col 42), essentially 'join[ing] in a row which they [did] not wholly understand' (House of Commons, 1989a: cols 35–6). In support of the Secretary of State, Conservative MPs went on the offensive, claiming that the 'BMA ha[d] lost much good will as a result of its campaign' (House of Commons, 1989a: col 1064) and 'malign propaganda' (House of Commons, 1989a: cols 1068–9).

Labour rallied around the BMA and issued a warning to Clarke that when 'get[ting] into such a ferocious rhetorical state about the propaganda spread by the BMA, he should be more careful, because he must [have been] spending hundreds of millions of pounds of taxpayers' money on putting his case' (House of Commons, 1989a: col 45).

The BMA called Clarke a 'bulldozer', accused him of ignoring medical advice, and rejected the proposal (Greener, 2009). Thatcher was also depicted in posters as a giant steamroller. The BMA pointed out that the issue of under-funding had been ignored and a damaging fragmentation of the NHS was underway (*BMJ*, 1989).

During the three-day parliamentary hearings on the Second Reading of the Community and Care Bill, the BMA's leadership and its stance against the reform were discussed in over 20 instances. Clarke 'never understood why the BMA opposed the proposal, as [he] felt it was on the wrong side of the barricade. The BMA [was] represent[ing] GPs in particular and it should have recommended to the Government a system that placed funds in the hands of GPs and gave them more influence over how resources are deployed' (House of Commons, 1989b: col 503).

However, the medical profession was adamant: the reform would 'destroy the comprehensive nature of the existing service' (House of Commons, 1989b: col 682). The Royal Colleges emphasised that there was 'no evidence that any of these radical proposals [would] improve patient care or patient access to care' (House of Commons, 1989b: col 1265). The former President of the Royal College of Surgeons, Lord Smith, stated that professional medical bodies 'regret[ted] the Secretary of State's refusal to debate with them his intentions before producing the Bill' (House of Commons, 1989b: col 1309).

The NHS and Community Care Bill passed in 1990, aided by Clarke's dogged determination not to balk under pressure from the medical profession (Ham, 2009), and came into effect in April 1991. Clarke paid a price, however, from the deterioration of relations between the Department of Health and the medical profession. He was eventually replaced by William Waldegrave, who favoured a more conciliatory approach to the development of an internal market, which some saw as a 'muddle between what was metaphor and what was reality' (quoted in Ham, 2000: 30).

In Waldegrave's view, 'it's not a market in that people don't go bust and make profits and all that, but it's using market-like mechanisms to provide better information' (Waldegrave, 1991: 636). As the medical profession's cooperation was needed to implement the reform, government sought to move beyond confrontation (Greener and Harrington, 2014).

Labour in power: (re)engineering consensus, 1997–2010

Back in power after nearly 20 years and with a substantial majority, the Labour government headed by Prime Minister Tony Blair issued a White Paper

(Secretary of State for Health, 1997) asserting the importance of healthcare professionals in running the NHS. It promised a quieter time in terms of change. It also signalled a return to a pre-Thatcher approach to change that was more inclusive, participatory and consensual (Baggott, 2015).

During this period, the medical profession accepted the need for reform and was more willing to work in cooperation with the State (Greener, 2009). The government wanted 'a system based on partnership and driven by performance' (Secretary of State for Health, 1997: 10), where 'what counts is what works' and 'modernisation' was the main goal (Ham, 2009). GP fundholding was immediately abolished, but the structure of the internal market was preserved and adapted, with a transition towards longer-term contracts, emphasis on partnership and less bureaucracy (Powell, 1998).

The first major policy intervention was the creation of Primary Care Groups (PCGs), which incorporated all family doctors and community nurses and offered them more freedom to allocate resources at local level (Ham, 2009). PCGs expected the medical profession to assume collective responsibility for overseeing the activities of other doctors, something that GPs had always opposed on the grounds of independence and autonomy (Klein, 2013).

GPs were also required to exercise checks on one another's expenditure to avoid overspending and recognise the scarcity of resources at collective level. The BMA had opposed GP fundholding, but in this instance acquiesced to the reform package, despite the fact that it included a number of measures that limited medical autonomy (Klein, 2013).

From 1948 to 1997, all GPs provided services according to a single contract negotiated with government. This changed with the NHS (Primary Care) Act, approved in 1997 right before Labour took power. It considered that the existing standard contract for General Medical Services (GMS) did not provide sufficient flexibility to serve all communities. A new Personal Medical Services (PMS) contract was thus introduced, which instead of being attached to individual GPs, referred to a group or a practice and included a defined package of services.

PMS contracts were negotiated locally rather than nationally to better reflect local needs and included criteria for service quality. Both the medical profession and the government had an interest in changing contractual arrangements. GPs wanted to reduce the amount of services they were required to provide to an essential core, gain flexibility and get rid of the obligation for 24-hour cover. The government wanted to improve access and quality of care and achieve a more varied skill mix in general practice.

In June 2001, GPs threatened to resign unless a more favourable agreement was put forth. Secretary of State for Health, Alan Milburn, decided to not engage in open dispute and instead let the NHS Confederation (the body representing NHS providers) handle negotiations. These inexperienced negotiators ended up drafting a contract that cost more and delivered somewhat less than expected (Rivett, 1998).

Ratified by the Health and Social Care Act 2003, the new contract relied on a complicated structure of incentives with nearly 150 indicators. The *BMJ* described it as 'more complex than the Minotaur's Labyrinth' (Smith, 2003). The contract was eventually accompanied by the introduction of two other forms of contract, one for services provided by Primary Care Trusts (PCTs, which succeeded PCGs) and one for privately owned practices.

Unbeknownst to the medical profession, the introduction of these new contractual forms meant that GPs lost their monopoly over service provision: people were now able to access private healthcare providers (Pollock et al, 2007). A few doctors raised this point to the BMA during negotiations, but they did not take it up.

Changes were also in the works for hospital specialist contracts, which, since 1948, comprised a fixed salary and bonus payments. The main distinction was between specialists working full-time or part-time for the NHS: the former could dedicate a maximum 10 per cent of their time to private practice while the latter had no such limit. The government and the medical profession agreed that the contract was inadequate and needed substantial modifications, but negotiations became confrontational (Klein, 2013).

The government and NHS managers sought increased control over specialists, particularly in relation to private practice. They also recognised the need to increase the number of specialists and simplify their pay scale by bringing together fixed and bonus amounts. The specialists welcomed some of the government's proposals, but were concerned about the introduction of appraisal systems and different job plans. The BMA perceived the proposal as a 'vicious attack' on the profession (Rivett, 1998).

Professional representatives engaged for nearly two years in negotiations that would eventually produce a more favourable financial arrangement in return for greater flexibility. However, negotiators on both sides misunderstood what junior doctors and specialists were looking for, and the proposal was rejected.

Representatives of the medical profession put forward a new contract proposal, with modest changes. Significantly, it eliminated 'the excessive and inappropriate managerial control' that, according to BMA representative Dr Paul Miller, was 'the sticking point' in the previous proposal (Kmietowicz, 2003). In October 2003, the deal was ratified with a small majority.

The contract was far more expensive than predicted, with consultants paid 25 per cent more on average than before for the same number of hours. As a result, some provider organisations ran into difficulties (NAO, 2007). The BMA concluded that agreeing to the new contract conditions 'was like taking a candy from a baby' (quoted in Klein, 2013: 237).

During this period, several serious cases of medical malpractice emerged, including in children's heart surgery at Bristol Royal Infirmary, the Royal Liverpool Children's Hospital and Alder Hey, and, most infamously, the murders by a Yorkshire GP, Dr Harold Shipman (Smith, 2002). The Bristol case in particular revealed a collective institutional failure at professional level. Professional self-regulation only worked effectively (but frequently retroactively) when the General Medical Council (GMC) stepped in as a measure of last resort.

The medical profession was under pressure to strengthen its system of accountability. The Secretary of State for Health decided to launch a public inquiry and the medical profession retreated into a defensive stance, accepting an unprecedented degree of scrutiny (Klein, 2013). Improving quality of care became the centrepiece of the policy agenda, with the government implicitly acknowledging that self-regulation was not sufficient to guarantee high standards (Ham, 2009).

Fully recognising the gravity of the situation, the President of the GMC, Sir Donald Irvine, stated that there was a need to redefine what it meant to be a medical professional and advocated a more active role for professional bodies (Irvine, 1999). The State's interventionist approach was accepted by the Royal Colleges and the GMC, which agreed to introduce revalidation processes for medical professionals. Collegial professional control survived, but only by giving up a considerable degree of individual professional autonomy (Klein, 2013).

A further twist in the regulatory role of the GMC came after the Shipman Inquiry, led by Chief Medical Officer Sir Liam Donaldson. In a further sign of distrust in professional self-regulation (Chief Medical Officer, 2006), the report recommended that members of the GMC no longer be elected by the medical profession, but instead be chosen by an independent body (the Appointments Commission). Importantly, there was little opposition to this proposal from the medical profession, partly because doctors had 'once more (had) their mouth stuffed with gold' in the new contracts, and partly because they sensed that the battle for autonomy had already been lost in the 1980s (Greener, 2006: 660).

Clinical governance was also introduced (Secretary of State for Health, 1998) and required providers to adopt systems for controlling medical performance. Clinical standards became National Service Frameworks, with compulsory participation by all doctors. Doctors were increasingly required to disclose and discuss their mistakes and participate in improving service areas with problems (Greener, 2009). According to Salter (2004: 140), the government had intruded on 'medical territory and the profession was ill prepared' to object.

Towards the end of the 1990s, the Labour government became increasingly dissatisfied with marginal gains in waiting lists, improvements in quality and organisational change in the system (Greener, 2009). In 1999, a new semi-autonomous organisation – the National Institute for Health and Care Excellence (NICE) – was created, with a mandate to evaluate existing and new treatments and to decide which ones should be paid for by the public purse. NICE therefore became the national rationing body for both medicines and treatments.

Another semi-autonomous organisation was set up to inspect the activity of healthcare organisations – the Commission for Health Improvement (known as the Care Quality Commission, CQC, after 2009). This body quickly introduced a wide-ranging programme of clinical governance reviews in order to monitor and improve provider services, from risk management and clinical audit to information use. It later became responsible for inspecting the private healthcare sector as well (Ham, 2009). This ramping up of control reinforced the managerial narrative in interactions between the State and the medical profession, with the former demanding ever-greater accountability from doctors to their employers and professional bodies (Greener, 2009).

By autumn 1999, it became clear that the NHS was heading toward financial crisis (Rivett, 1998). In what was defined as 'the most expensive breakfast in history' – referring to statements Prime Minister Blair made on a morning TV show (Klein, 2013) – in March 2000 extra money was allocated to the NHS on condition that the service modernise and that the medical profession commit to working towards its redesign.

In July 2000, a new 10-year strategy –*The NHS Plan* – was published (Secretary of State for Health, 2000). Secretary of State for Health Alan Milburn wanted to create 'a big-tent coalition of support' for reform goals (Alvarez-Rosete and Mays, 2014: 634). The plan was the result of work by a number of Modernisation Action Teams focusing on different challenges faced by the NHS (Platt, 1998). Their composition was broad and comprised NHS staff, patient representatives, professional associations, academics and other sectors (Ham, 2009). Team members were invited as experts and not as formal representatives of different groups. In this way, Milburn sought to achieve inclusivity while pre-empting opposition (Alvarez-Rosete and Mays, 2014).

The Modernisation Action Teams were favourably received within the NHS and were seen as the 'largest ever public consultation exercise on healthcare services' (McIver, 2000). The medical profession enthusiastically embraced its role in the policy formulation process (Rivett, 1998). The presidents of the Royal Colleges and the chair of the BMA endorsed the government's efforts to modernise the NHS in the Preface to the White Paper that resulted from this work. The BMA shared the view that the service was underfunded and that shortages of doctors and nurses had to be tackled.

The NHS Plan was approved, and in its launch, the government took pains to garner professional consensus and mobilise doctors' support (Klein,

2013). In contrast to their vehement opposition to the Clarke reforms of the Thatcher era, professional associations were supportive (Rivett, 1998), although their involvement in implementing the modernisation reforms was less clear (Alvarez-Rosete and Mays, 2014).

The reform package introduced for the first time a new system of performance ratings, exposing service providers to wider scrutiny by making ratings public with a traffic light approach and then star ratings. Organisations that met national standards received extra funding and greater autonomy. Conversely, failing trusts faced the prospect of being 'franchised' to managers of other successful NHS trusts or to private sector providers (Greener, 2009). Managers were held accountable for their trust's failings, and could lose their jobs if they underperformed (Dawson and Dargie, 2002). Unsurprisingly, this command-and-control approach was unpopular within the NHS and attracted much criticism (Klein, 2013).

The reform also introduced a market-like system of payment for providers called 'payment by results' (Department of Health, 2002). Providers no longer received block funding, but were paid in relation to the activities they conducted, based on fixed tariffs (or Health Resource Groups) adjusted for local market conditions. These rewarded busier Hospital Trusts. These measures represented fundamental changes in the functioning of the NHS, but the medical profession showed little interest in engaging with them.

Moreover, to achieve greater plurality of provision and shorten waiting lists, the Labour government opened up the service to private and not-for-profit sectors. The aim was to increase private sector access to the NHS market in areas of need (for example, testing), but also to promote the development of public–private partnerships (Ham, 2009). The Labour Party was not entirely united behind greater private sector involvement and the medical profession was also on the fence. The BMA feared it would lead to wholesale privatisation (Rivett, 1998).

Nevertheless, from that moment on, the private sector became an integral, albeit small, player in the provision of NHS services (Greener, 2005). Capacity increased and the State became less reliant on NHS medical professionals in the delivery of services. Furthermore, a new organisational form, the Foundation Trust, was introduced in 2002 with the aim of giving high-performing providers more autonomy and freedom in service design and the allocation of resources.

Further reforms were announced in the *NHS Improvement Plan* published in June 2004 (Secretary of State for Health, 2004). Among other objectives, the focus was to further reduce waiting times and enable patients to consult any provider meeting standards set by the regulator, who would be paid on the basis of the national tariff system (Ham, 2009). The government also wanted to improve the health of the population and proposed transferring the commissioning role from PCTs to individual GP practices. However, this proposal met with concerns from trade unions that saw it as a potential precursor to privatisation, and it was eventually dropped (Ham, 2009). Following an independent review, the number of PCTs was cut in half (from 303 to 152), essentially to create bigger organisations that could match the size of healthcare providers.

Towards the end of the Blair period, doctors complained of heavy workloads and the pace of reforms driven by the modernisation agenda. Blair infuriated the BMA by suggesting that it was part of the 'forces of conservatism' working against public services reform. Hostility increased after the adoption of more pronounced market-style policies in the NHS. However, some commentators noted that the BMA lost its power to influence government in the latter years of the Blair government (Baggott, 2015).

The Royal Colleges, on the other hand, appeared to consolidate their position, and the Royal College of Physicians in particular became increasingly influential (Sheard and Donaldson, 2006; Baggott, 2015). This was potentially due to their willingness to work with government behind closed doors. Conversely, the BMA, which consistently and publicly challenged the government, was held at arm's length. There was a sense that the 'insider status' of the medical profession (and especially of the BMA) in policy-making had progressively weakened (Alvarez-Rosete and Mays, 2008).

Gordon Brown took over from Blair as Prime Minister in June 2007, and was less inclined to market-based approaches and more predisposed to empowering citizens, fostering a new professionalism and providing better leadership (Ham, 2009). Government objectives became explicit after the completion of a review of the service conducted by a prominent clinician, Lord Ara Darzi, who was, unusually, also given a position within government.

The Darzi review involved more than 2,000 doctors and other healthcare professionals. Its report, *High Quality Care for All*, was published in October 2008, and emphasised the need to improve the quality of care and patient safety (Secretary of State for Health, 2008). This was to be achieved through a bottom-up strategy, where staff would lead improvement efforts across the service and thoroughly engage in the implementation process (Klein, 2013). This high-profile call for greater clinical leadership in the management of the NHS became a staple for the years to come.

The coalition period and a return to conflict, 2010–20

The run-up to the 2010 General Election saw the traditional declarations from the main political parties of commitment towards the NHS and its founding principles (Klein, 2013). Labour lost the election by a handful of seats and a new Conservative–Liberal Democrat coalition government was formed. The economy was still reeling from the effects of the global financial crisis of 2007–08 and public finances had to be tightened.

In July 2010 (just 60 days after the election), the new Secretary of State for Health, Andrew Lansley, published the White Paper *Equity and Excellence: Liberating the NHS* (Secretary of State for Health, 2010). His proposals were based on a draft he had written for the Conservative Party while acting as Shadow Health Secretary during the Liberal reign, and built on the principles of increasing competition and devolving decision-making (Lansley, 2005). Liberating the NHS included an unexpectedly radical set of ideas.

Central to Lansley's proposals was a substantive shift in power and accountability. Additionally, he wanted to reduce the scope for change by future governments. Officials in the Department of Health warned him that a large-scale reorganisation was not feasible at a time of mounting financial pressures, but he pressed ahead regardless (Timmins, 2012).

Among the main organisational changes proposed in Lansley's White Paper was the replacement of PCTs by a consortia of budget-holding GPs – Clinical Commissioning Groups (CCGs) – which would receive funding according to the size and composition of their local populations; a commitment to cut management costs by 45 per cent; and the transformation of all NHS providers into Foundation Trusts. A new body was also introduced, the NHS Commissioning Board (later renamed NHS England), with responsibility for national and regional specialist services, but also a broad executive function over the whole NHS separated from the Department of Health.

Prior to the White Paper's release, Lansley engaged in conversations with primary care representatives such as the National Association of Primary Care and the NHS Alliance, but their input was not well reflected in the resulting plan (Timmins, 2012). Medical doctors were surprised and consternated by *Liberating the NHS*, partly due to the scale and speed at which organisational changes were meant to take place, and partly because its implications were not immediately clear. Furthermore, the new coalition government had just vowed to stop top-down reorganisations of the NHS (HM Government, 2010).

Criticism of the Health Secretary mounted and gained momentum after the details of the plan were made explicit in the parliamentary Bill in January 2011. The BMA thought the Bill was 'a massive gamble' and likened Lansley's proposals to the Thatcher reforms. The BMA stated it did not support 'the direction taken by the NHS in England in recent years, which is continued, and indeed accelerated by the proposals set out in the White Paper' (BMA, 2010: 1). Among other critiques, the BMA specifically targeted the 'active promotion of a market approach' and the goal of opening up local areas to 'any willing provider' (BMA, 2010: 1). This was in line with its opposition to Clarke's reforms and 'anti-privatisation campaign' over the years (Timmins, 2012).

The BMA maintained its opposition throughout the parliamentary process and, towards the end, was joined by the RCGP. College Chair Dr Clare Gerada claimed that 'the reorganisation represented no less than the privatisation of the NHS' (quoted in Greener and Harrington, 2014), and that the proposals would be 'the end of the NHS as we know it' (quoted in Timmins, 2012: 74). The other Royal Colleges did not immediately assume an openly antagonistic position, but increasingly criticised the reform package. The National Association for Primary Care, on the other hand, supported the reforms on the grounds that they gave GPs the power to purchase goods for the benefit of patients (Greener and Harrington, 2014). Similarly, the NHS Alliance considered that GP commissioning 'was emancipating – all that we could have asked for' (quoted in Timmins, 2012: 70).

The Bill was presented to Parliament for its Second Reading on 31 January 2011. Once again, Labour MPs became spokespeople for medical professional bodies. Many statements relating the 'disquiet and concern among health professionals about the speed and scale of the reforms outlined in the Bill' were put forward during discussions. A declaration from the Royal Society of Physicians was quoted, saying that '[a]chieving both efficiency savings and reorganisation simultaneously [would] be an unprecedented challenge for both commissioners and providers'.

The BMA warned that: 'failed consortia [would be] bought up on the cheap by foreign companies and see bits of the NHS run from abroad' (House of Commons, 2011: cols 691–2). Furthermore, the lack of consultation and consensus around the Bill was understood as a 'lack of attention paid to stakeholders' concerns' (House of Lords, 2011: col 694). Eventually, in March 2011, the BMA formally requested that the Bill be dropped. This went against the advice of BMA Chair, Dr Meldrum, and a special meeting was convened to discuss his position (Timmins, 2012).

Groups such as the NHS Confederation expressed concerns about the vagueness of some of the policy aims, including the role and functions of CCGs (Klein, 2013). The House of Commons Health Committee, chaired by a former Conservative Health Secretary, Stephen Dorrell, also questioned several points of the legislation (House of Commons Health Committee, 2010). Some Conservative MPs believed that the Bill was one of the greatest mistakes made by the party, calling it a 'huge strategic error' (quoted in Smyth et al, 2014).

In an unprecedented move, in March 2011, Prime Minister David Cameron and Liberal Democrat Deputy Prime Minister Nick Clegg requested a halt in the legislative process of the Bill. Professional and public opinion was openly against the reforms, and Cameron sought to protect his position by taking charge and initiating a 'listening exercise' (Klein, 2013). A consultation was conducted by the NHS Future Forum (essentially an ad hoc Commission), and led to important changes in the reform package.

The Forum was chaired by a GP, Professor Steve Field, and around a third of its members were medical professionals. The profession as a whole was then widely consulted. The final report related 'deep seated concern', but did not outright reject Lansley's reform package (NHS Future Forum, 2011). The Forum did, however, recommend mitigating changes that would, in some critics' estimation, lead to the fragmentation and privatisation of the NHS (Klein, 2013). The review was conducted at breakneck speed, and the NHS Future Forum report was published in June 2011. The government accepted almost all proposed changes to the Bill (Secretary of State for Health, 2011).

Despite some major concessions, however, the criticism of those opposed to the Bill did not stop. At the beginning of the 2012, the government had completely lost the chance of bringing healthcare professionals on board. Both medical and nursing professional associations were adamantly opposed to competition and concerned about the possibility that access to healthcare services would be reduced (Godlee, 2012).

At the BMA's Annual Conference, members again opposed the recommendation of the Association's leadership and demanded that the Bill be withdrawn as it had remained 'a monster of a lipstick' (Timmins, 2012). When the Bill was introduced for a second time in Parliament, the medical profession had already mobilised its community: 'There [had been] an overwhelming call for [Members of the House of Lords] to stop the Bill from the royal colleges, the professions, doctors, nurses, thousands of health workers, patients and, indeed, non-patients' (House of Lords, 2011: col 1482). In fact, 'the level of concern about [the] Bill [was] virtually unprecedented' (House of Lords, 2011: col 1529).

Some members of the House, however, had the impression that the medical profession was lobbying in favour of the status quo because of 'vested interests in the BMA and elsewhere in keeping things unchanged and unchallenged. ... At the same time, a nostalgic view of the NHS was prevail[ing] which [was] anti-business' (House of Lords, 2011: col 1511).

Lords supporting the reforms contended that the government had encouraged the profession to cooperate and had actively invited medical practitioners into the negotiating space: a 'series of fascinating seminars about all aspects of [the] Bill ... [and] the opportunity to question think tanks, Royal Colleges and senior civil servants was made available to all Peers and was taken up by many' (House of Lords, 2011: col 1485). Objections to the legislation were thereby put down to a lack of unity and contested leadership within the medical profession.

Some of the Liberal Democrat and Conservative Lords even argued that '[a] lot of GPs [were] enthusiastic and well informed, despite the unbending criticism of the Bill by the chairman of the council of the Royal College of General Practitioners' (House of Lords, 2011: col 1542). They also argued that since '[t]he White Paper called for clinical leadership ... [it was] time for the medical profession to stand up and be counted' (House of Lords, 2011: col 1514). Eventually, a letter signed by 400 public health doctors against the legislation forced the House of Lords to adopt amendments.

In January 2012, at a joint meeting, the 20 Royal Colleges failed to agree on a common statement, but the main professional journals produced an unprecedented joint editorial condemning the Bill. In February, the BMA asked for the Bill's full withdrawal and a campaign among professionals led the Royal Colleges to finally reach a consensus position rejecting the reforms (Timmins, 2012).

A subsequent meeting between the government and a selected group of medical professionals failed to achieve any breakthroughs. However, the coalition government closed ranks and the Bill was finally sent back to the House of Commons for approval. In March 2012, Parliament approved the Health and Social Care Bill and with it, possibly one of the most complex programmes of change in NHS history (Klein, 2013).

Beyond the quagmire of Lansley's reforms, the NHS faced a prolonged period of cutbacks and service pressures (The King's Fund, 2015). Fiscal austerity dominated public finances and the NHS budget was cut in real terms over this period. In the 2015 Treasury Budget, Chancellor George Osborne announced a four-year pay freeze for the whole of the public sector. The BMA accused the government of not finding other means of making NHS finances more sustainable (Iacobucci, 2015).

Lansley did not survive his reforms, and in September 2012 was replaced by Jeremy Hunt, while Simon Stevens replaced David Nicholson as Chief Executive of NHS England. Stevens had progressive views on the NHS, including on competition. Under his leadership, NHS England published the *Five Year Forward View* (5YFV) (NHS England, 2014). A key part of the new plan was the integration of healthcare and social care services, relying on greater collaboration among providers.

Like the 2000 *NHS Plan*, the 5YFV was well received by the main NHS bodies such as Monitor, the CQC, Public Health England and NICE, which had been actively involved in discussions around the plan. The medical profession was more cautious. Some expressed enthusiasm (Iacobucci, 2014). Others, especially front-line clinicians, felt that the plan lacked details on how greater integration would be achieved through an increasing role of CCGs and the rationalisation of acute care services (Cruickshank and Jenkins, 2014).

To the surprise of many commentators who believed another minority government was on the cards, the 2015 General Election gave the Conservative Party a small majority in Parliament and David Cameron was confirmed as Prime Minister. In the quest for service integration, a new organisational form was introduced toward the end of 2015: Sustainability and Transformation Plans (STPs).

STPs were meant to fill the leadership vacuum left at regional level by the abolition of strategic health authorities (SHAs) (Health and Social Care Act, 2012) and, rather unusually, were introduced without a specific legal framework or formal accountability structure. The main goal was to reduce use of acute and community hospitals and adapt the delivery of specialised services to local needs.

The BMA appeared to approach STPs with an open mind, and recognised that STPs might have a role to play in adapting services to local needs. However, they expressed reservations over the lack of consultation of medical professionals. In a survey of its members, the BMA found that more than 60 per cent had not been consulted and more than a third had never heard of STPs.

One of the main criticisms of STPs was their perceived lack of transparency and accountability in the redesign of services. The Head of the BMA, Dr Mark Porter, was quoted as saying: 'Given the scale of the savings required in each area, there is a real risk that these transformation plans will be used as a cover for delivering cuts, starving services of resource and patients of vital care' (quoted in Siddique, 2016).

Similarly, the President of the Royal College of Emergency Medicine lamented a lack of engagement with the medical profession and gave a stark warning over plans that appeared 'seriously alarming and potentially catastrophic'. The Royal College of Physicians supported the policy in principle, but cautioned that general practice and individuals needed to be at the core of the plans. Criticism from the College became more open when it appeared that some STPs planned to reduce GP numbers and prioritise acute Hospital Trusts (RCP, 2017). However, the NHS seemed to be in a relatively tranquil place.

Two events in 2016 completely changed the outlook for the government and the NHS. First was the Brexit Referendum ordered by Cameron, which unexpectedly resulted in a win, by a very small majority, for the Leave side wanting to extricate the UK from the European Union (EU). Cameron resigned and Theresa May became Prime Minister in July 2016. Brexit remained a major distraction throughout her premiership and beyond. The second event was internal to the NHS and was related to a catastrophic decision made by Secretary of State for Health Jeremy Hunt to unilaterally change the contractual agreement with junior doctors.

The Conservative government aimed to address the risk of poor quality of hospital care at weekends. A high-profile report published by the *Journal of the Royal Society of Medicine* showed mortality rates spiking outside normal workweek hours as well as immediately after newly qualified doctors started their first post (Freemantle et al, 2012). The report recommended having some specialists on site at all times, which required changes in working pattern. Interestingly, the Royal College of Physicians was in favour of a seven-day working week, which also figured in the 5YFV (RCP, 2013). Hunt wanted to increase pay during the week and reduce it at the weekend to dissuade junior doctors from being available in place of consultants.

In September 2015, Hunt proposed a contract that abolished overtime pay between 7am and 10pm, apart from Sundays. Refusing to enter into negotiations, the BMA pointed out that the proposal would increase working hours while effectively cutting pay by 40 per cent (BMA, 2015). Hunt refused to back down. The BMA responded by announcing its intention to hold a members' vote, and a survey of junior doctors showed that 70 per cent were considering leaving the NHS if the contract was approved (Campbell, 2015).

A slightly modify contract proposal was tabled in November 2015, but the Chair of the BMA Junior Doctors' Committee, Dr Johann Malawana, rejected it, saying 'the proposals on pay, not for the first time, appear to be misleading. The increase in basic pay would be offset by changes to pay for unsocial hours, devaluing the vital work junior doctors do at evenings and weekends' (quoted in Campbell, 2015). The BMA took offense at Hunt's unwillingness to compromise and held another members' vote on 5 November 2015, with job action anticipated in December. On 24 December, Malawana issued an ultimatum: progress in negotiations or job action (*The Guardian*, 2015).

On 12 January 2016, for the first time in the history of the NHS, junior doctors undertook a day-long general strike across England. They withdrew routine care provision again on 10 February and, on 26 April, suspended both emergency and routine care. A new contract was agreed by the BMA on 18 May, but in July, a robust majority (58 per cent) of junior doctors once again voted against the deal. Unmoved, Hunt declared that the contract would be introduced over 12 months starting in October 2016.

Enraged by this further act of disrespect, and supported by the lobby group Justice for Health, a number of junior doctors brought the matter to court. A judicial review was ordered but on 28 September, Justice Green ruled against the junior doctors' claim that the contract was unlawful. He nonetheless expressed sympathy for the junior doctors in his opening remarks, echoing the broader population's support for NHS workers:

> The issue of the proposed new contract generates strong feelings. Evidence before the Court demonstrates the level of disenchantment which many junior doctors feel about their working conditions within the NHS. Much of this sentiment is of a general nature and whilst undoubtedly heartfelt is not always of direct relevance to the quite specific legal issues that I have to decide. (*Justice for Health Ltd, R vs The Secretary of State for Health*, 2016)

Unshaken by the judicial defeat, the BMA announced further strikes but did not, in the end, follow through on this threat. In June 2019, more favourable contract conditions were finally secured by the BMA with an 8.2 per cent pay increase over four years.

In July 2019, Dr Scarlett Hallett, a junior doctor at the Derby Hospitals NHS Foundation Trust, brought a claim against her employer related to the calculation of break time in her contract. She first lost her case in High Court (2018) but won in the Court of Appeals (2019). The breach of contract was estimated to have resulted in £250,000 unpaid supplementary pay for each doctor, a cost that was qualified by the court as 'potentially significant' for the NHS to reimburse (*Hallett vs Derby Hospitals*, 2018).

The ruling constituted a test case for the interpretation of doctors' employment contracts and provisions relating to their working conditions. It also signalled that medical doctors were prepared to take a new approach to managing their relationship with the State. While differences had previously been dealt with outside legal structures, including cases relating to specialist doctors and their NHS employers (Kahn-Freund, 1972), the judicial review sparked by junior doctors in 2016, as well as the more recent test case, revealed a willingness to depart from that tradition.

Part 2: Analysis of the NHS England case

Creating the NHS, pre-1948

The influence of context: drivers and shapers of medical politics

The historical context of the 1940s provided fertile ground for social reforms in England, including a strong political and societal mandate for better healthcare. During the Second World War, the government had clearly stated its intention to establish a nationwide comprehensive health service following recommendations of the inter-war Beveridge Report (Beveridge, 1942). Bipartisan parliamentary support for the recommendations reflected the collective thirst for a national solution.

The medical profession shared this priority, recognising that existing healthcare provision was deficient in quality and especially in terms of coverage. As described earlier in this chapter, the BMA nevertheless remained non-committal to the Beveridge plan, preferring to build on the existing insurance scheme and keep doctors outside government's direct sphere of influence.

Individual ambition also played a key role in the creation of a unified healthcare system in the UK. In particular, the appointment to the Department of Health of Aneurin Bevan, famously untethered to party lines and in favour of unifying hospital management, was an important factor in the build-up to 1948. His determination to face opposition from the medical profession was instrumental to the enactment of the National Health Service Bill in 1946.

Bevan did, however, have to deal with opposition from GPs and make a number of compromises. The pre-NHS referral system was demand-led and gave GPs an advantageous position over specialists and hospitals, whose income depended on GP referrals. In the NHS arrangement, GPs lost this position of power and therefore expected the BMA to protect their interests.

Strategies used by the protagonists to accommodate and deal with the evolving context

The medical profession trod cautiously around the two principles of universal and free provision that were at the centre of the reform proposal. The 1944 White Paper emphasised the government's willingness to establish a working relationship with the medical profession and in particular, with GPs, who were more exposed to potential radical changes. Consequently, the government never seriously contemplated disrupting the traditional separation between primary care, acute care and community health services, as this would compromise the collaboration of the medical profession.

Doctors saw a national system as a threat to their autonomy and earnings. Even in the heady spirit of 1942, the BMA approved universal access to healthcare by only a small majority (BMA, 1942), and their approval was linked to assurance that GPs would not fall under the control of local authorities. Caught between the political and societal support for a public healthcare system and the need to protect its members, the BMA maintained a generally ambivalent position throughout the negotiations. Hostility towards Bevan represented a badge of honour, but to an extent this was worn as an 'opportunity to wash their hands over some of the compromises they were accepting' rather than representing concrete opposition to his plans (Klein, 2013: 12).

The government was aware that refusing all the demands of the medical profession would have killed the legislation. For example, the President of the Royal College of Physicians, Lord Moran, made it clear that doctors would only entertain discussions on the NHS if hospitals were not placed under the control of local authorities, so this option was never seriously considered (Titmuss, 1958).

Breaking with tradition, Bevan tactically decided against prior consultation with the whole of the medical profession on the reform proposals. Allegedly to privilege democratic scrutiny, proposals were presented to the Houses of Parliament before being submitted to the scrutiny of doctors (Rintala, 2003). Unconvinced about the motives underpinning this approach, the BMA perceived Bevan as an uncompromising figure who was intentionally trying to gain leverage in negotiations.

Bevan's approach was indeed subtle. He engaged in secret conversations with a few leaders of the medical profession in an attempt to find common ground (Rintala, 2003). Hospital doctors were his preferred partners because their representative bodies, the Royal Colleges, could make decisions without consulting members, unlike the BMA (Honigsbaum, 1989). Fundamentally, the government's strategy was to split the medical profession and strike a deal with doctors involved in hospital medicine.

This less formal style of consultation suited hospital specialists. By offering them generous financial conditions and operational concessions, including a new system of awards and distinctions, Bevan was able to secure the support of what he perceived as the most influential group of medical professionals (Jones, 2014). On the other hand, GPs received far fewer concessions and perceived the reform as a threat to their self-employed status. Bevan dithered with, but eventually abandoned, the idea of having GPs work under local authorities.

To bring the BMA on board, the government had to engage in complex negotiations and was ultimately forced to provide assurance that GP autonomy, freedom of work and self-administration would not be challenged (Pater, 1981). Squeezed between broad support for the proposed NHS and the firm demands of GPs, the BMA eventually approved the plan on the condition that GPs would not be forced into becoming salaried employees of local authorities (Honigsbaum, 1989).

Implications for medical politics and health reforms

The final agreement between the two main protagonists legitimised and institutionalised the 'double bed' relationship between the State and the medical profession (Klein, 2013). The State – assuming the role of sole employer (purchaser of services) – was willing to give the medical profession an almost 'free hand' in running health services within a budget set by the State in return for their support for reforms. The two entered into a binding agreement ('concordat') where the needs of one would be balanced by the demands of the other.

The resulting relationship was characterised by accommodation of the interests and needs of these two main protagonists. The nationalisation of hospitals not only gave specialists great power and control within their domain, but also flipped their relationship with GPs. Prior to 1948, specialists had to rely on GP referrals for patients (and thus earnings). This form of dependency disappeared when specialists became salaried employees.

While not especially pleased with this less favourable arrangement, GPs, like specialists, were able to maintain their autonomy. This phase of reform revealed that the stance taken by the medical profession was far from homogenous (Klein, 2013), and this difference in needs and interests periodically re-emerged in the years that followed.

Importantly, the 'double bed' relationship meant that the medical profession rarely questioned the legitimacy of the NHS. When it did, the critique was mainly directed towards weaknesses in the funding model rather than the principle of a universal public healthcare system. After 1948, GPs positioned themselves as the guardians of the system and repeatedly challenged reform proposals on the principle that these would negatively affect the values underpinning the NHS (Crinson, 1998).

Additionally, the mutual dependency between the State and medical profession led to the creation of an informal 'policy community' involving the Department of Health, the Royal Colleges and the BMA (Smith, 1993). For many years, health policy was designed through an adaptive and gradual process built on broad consensus.

30 years of 'consensus', 1948–79

The influence of context: drivers and shapers of medical politics

Like many other countries, the UK experienced a 'golden age' of welfare politics between the end of the war and the 1970s. The two dominant political parties were in broad agreement over health policy in general and the organisation of the health service (Kavanagh and Morris, 1989), which enabled a (long) period of relative calm in the NHS (Greener, 2009). However, the real cost of running the NHS was miscalculated at the outset and supplementary funding was required (Public Records Office, 1948).

According to NHS architect Bevan, part of the increased cost was a direct consequence of 'a nationally owned and administered hospital service which will always involve a very considerable and expanding Exchequer outlay' (Public Records Office, 1950a). But he also pointed to doctors' 'too great a degree of control over hospital management committees', and lack of regard for financial limits (Public Records Office, 1950b). The endless debate over the allocation of finite resources and the most effective way to manage the service entered the mediated space.

Meanwhile, a schism was developing between the two branches of the medical profession. While hospital doctors accrued a number of benefits with the creation of the NHS, GPs suffered progressively worsening working and financial conditions. To make matters worse, GPs' representative body, the BMA, saw its influence diminish. The BMA had fought vigorously in the run-up to July 1948 for GP autonomy and, as a consequence, the government became less inclined to improve conditions in general practice, especially if this meant taking resources away from hospitals (Webster, 1988).

The prolonged era of increasing budgets for the NHS came to an end when the government faced a slowing economy and fiscal crises in the 1970s (Lowe,

1998). This brought to the fore the structural issues caused by the tripartite arrangement (organisationally separated primary, secondary and tertiary care functions), and emphasised the need for a significant reorganisation. The National Health Service Reorganisation Act 1973, which was eventually supported by the medical profession, involved significant restructuring of the NHS, but failed to solve many issues and generated new costs and low staff morale, the latter compounded by worsening living standards (Ham, 2009).

Strategies used by the protagonists to accommodate and deal with the evolving context

Developments in the 1970s confirmed GPs' misgivings about the original agreement struck between the BMA and Bevan, especially around working conditions and their status vis-à-vis specialists (Calnan and Gabe, 1991). According to *The Lancet*, 'on balance the effects of the [NHS] Act on [GP] practice have so far been for the worse and there is little evidence that its problems are being squarely faced' (Fox, 1950). The perception of inequality in relation to specialists was amplified when Lord Moran, President of the Royal College of Physicians, suggested that GPs were 'somewhat an inferior bunch' (quoted in Rivett, 1998: 163).

Despite opposition from the Royal Colleges, which were fearful of diluting their influence, the College of General Practitioners was created in 1952 and became an important conduit for GP demands. The BMA was struggling to act as an effective representative for family doctors as this conflicted with its ambition to provide a unified voice for the whole medical profession (Greener, 2009).

The crisis of representation also prompted the appearance of a breakaway General Practitioners' Association and increasing membership in the Medical Practitioners' Union. The proliferation of representative GP bodies seeded a more conflictual relationship with the State.

The 1960 Royal Commission report on Doctors' and Dentists' Remuneration, set up by Prime Minister Harold Macmillan, added fuel to the fire, as it highlighted growing disparities between factions of the medical profession and the need for a permanent review body to address medical compensation. Hospital specialists not only benefited from better financial conditions, but also had permanent control of management structures in hospitals and regional bodies (Greener, 2009).

The *BMJ* was filled with letters from disillusioned GPs (*BMJ*, 1963, 1964), and this widespread malaise culminated with the BMA publishing the *Charter for the Family Doctor Service* in 1965 (Cameron, 1965). The adoption a new GP contract in 1966 was only achieved after a complex round of negations, marked by GP resistance to giving full negotiating powers to their representatives (Loudon et al, 1998).

Tasked with conducting a 10-year review of the NHS, the high-profile 1962 Porritt Committee, set up as a collaborative effort between the government, the BMA and the Royal Colleges, recommended the unification of healthcare provision, with GPs taking a greater role in planning services (Medical Services Review Committee, 1962). However, the substantial new investment in the NHS following the review – endorsed by the medical profession – was directed exclusively towards acute care provision in a 10-year programme to modernise crumbling infrastructure.

Divisions between GPs and specialists aside, this period was an example of what could be achieved through collaboration between the government and the medical profession. However, despite this positive relationship between the two main actors, at the end of the 1960s faith in the effectiveness of a hospital-dominated health service began to wane. Managerial ideas started to crop up in discussions around the NHS, and the Conservative government brought in management consultants (McKinsey & Co.) to advise on changes that would mitigate doctors' control over hospital administration.

The medical profession discredited the applicability of management jargon and ideas to medical services (*BMJ*, 1969; *The Lancet*, 1971), and government capitulated. The reorganisation of 1974 not only failed to diminish the medical profession's control, but also actually expanded the role of doctors in running health services (Halcrow, 1989).

GPs had developed a stronger voice in 1965 with the *Charter for Family Doctors*, but their actions turned more confrontational when they joined forces with hospital specialists in the 1970s. Energised by a new-found sense of unity, the medical profession began using industrial action to obtain concessions from government. The junior doctors' strike of 1975 was actively promoted by medical unions, and especially by new more radical players such as the Medical Practitioners' Union. The Royal Colleges and the BMA were perceived by some as elitist and out of date (Greener, 2009).

Junior doctors formed their own association in 1966, which immediately campaigned to reduce pay differentials among specialists. In 1974, the body representing specialists (the Hospital Consultants' and Specialists' Association) led an unsuccessful court challenge against the BMA to obtain negotiating rights in labour disputes (Barnard and Lee, 1977). Representative pluralism was compromising the collective bargaining power of the medical profession (Klein, 2013). The pay settlement satisfied the demands of junior doctors, but irked the more experienced hospital specialists who benefited from the existing pay gap.

Additional turmoil was generated in 1974 when Health Secretary Barbara Castle announced an end to the practice of allowing privately paid beds in public hospitals. Coming at the same time as negotiations over a new specialists' contract, the pay beds dispute developed into a full-blown confrontation between the State and medical profession (Greener, 2009).

The BMA threw its weight behind the specialists, calling for strike action in July 1974; this was called off only when government accepted to return to the negotiating table (*BMJ*, 1974). This marked the first time in NHS history that hospital specialists were prepared to withhold services. The *BMJ* expressed dismay over what it saw as a decline in 'professional self-esteem' (*BMJ*, 1975).

The Cabinet had little appetite to fight specialists on this point. The Health Secretary was forced to concede to considerably better pay conditions (an increase of more than 30 per cent) and an arbitrated settlement resulted in just a limited reduction in specialists' use of private beds.

Implications for medical politics and healthcare reforms

This period had a major impact on the relationship between the State and the medical profession. GPs fought to maintain their status as independent contractors, while specialists argued for the preservation of their clinical freedom and privileges even as salaried employees. The power of the medical profession was openly acknowledged by the government, and civil servants highlighted in Parliament how 'the existence of clinical freedom undoubtedly reduces the ability of central authorities to determine objectives and priorities and to control individual facets of expenditure' (Expenditure Committee, 1971).

Still, the period up to the mid-1970s was characterised by a 'corporatist' relationship, with the protagonists jointly working at policy-making 'in smoked-filled rooms' (Moran, 1995). However, this was only true for one elite group in the medical profession, hospital specialists, who were given special access to the policy process in order to achieve 'engineered consensus' (Klein, 2013). In contrast, conflicts pitting GPs against the government over pay and status became commonplace.

The confrontations of the 1970s revealed that doctors were ready to openly show their mettle, but also that the State was increasingly prepared to take tough stances against the medical profession. The historical bargaining approach began to erode and the 'double bed' relationship grew frosty (Greener, 2009). Rapidly worsening public finances and confrontations over pay revealed underlying tensions and made agreement more difficult. Mutual dependency was less evident and the medical profession felt free to adopt (or threaten) more confrontational tactics such as strikes.

Similarly, this period saw increasing acrimony between doctor groups: GPs complained about the differential treatment of hospital doctors, junior doctors challenged their pay gap with experienced specialists, and specialists in turn complained about the erosion of their privileges within the profession (Klein, 2013). In consequence, the established voice of the profession, the BMA, experienced a crisis of representation that grew to the point that members demanded external scrutiny over its constitution and organisation (*BMJ*, 1972).

The Thatcher and Major era: consensual disagreement, 1979–97

The influence of context: drivers and shapers of medical politics

The starting point for this 18-year period under the Conservative government was the acknowledgement that, rather than unifying services and improving decision-making, the 1974 reorganisation had been costly in terms of NHS finances and staff morale (Royal Commission on the National Health Service, 1979). Sensing the opportunity for a decisive intervention, the new Thatcher government released the White Paper *Patient First* in 1979 (DHSS, 1979) following on recommendations of a Royal Commission to reduce bureaucracy in the NHS (Ham, 2009).

The medical profession saw merit in the idea of bringing services closer to patients (*BMJ*, 1980), but did not foresee the dramatic changes in store in the health policy arena. The government was eager to reduce public expenditure and provide more opportunity for the private sector to provide healthcare services. This triggered a predictable stand-off between the State and medical profession, with the former wanting to increase outputs through a range of market-oriented incentives, and the latter seeking to maintain constant growth of inputs into the NHS (Klein, 2013).

In the chaotic 1980s, changes were introduced via a series of somewhat disjointed policies rather than through a coherent programme of reforms (Ham, 2009). The reform that clearly marked the first half of the 1980s was the introduction of general management following the Griffiths report of 1983 (DHSS, 1983). Griffiths' observations about the NHS – many of which were shared by the medical profession (*BMJ*, 1983) – focused on NHS management's inability to use resources efficiently and tailor services around patient needs (Ham, 2009).

Buoyed by the report's recommendations, and despite the opposition of the medical profession, the government introduced a new cadre of general managers at all levels in the NHS. This move was highly disruptive of the 'double bed' relationship, with medical professionals losing their stranglehold on running the NHS.

The impact of underfunding the NHS became more apparent towards the end of the decade, marked by bed closures and a freeze on recruitment (NAHA, 1987). The government injected new funds but also initiated another wide-ranging review. It concluded that the funding model was adequate, but that drastic measures were needed because, as Thatcher stated (1993), 'the NHS had become a bottomless financial pit'. The 1989 White Paper *Working for Patients* announced the separation of purchasers and providers, with GPs taking on the purchaser role and competition installed between self-governing Hospital Trusts (Secretaries of State for Health, Wales, Northern Ireland, and Scotland, 1989).

Strategies used by the protagonists to accommodate and deal with the evolving context

The confrontational stance the medical profession developed in the 1970s persisted in the following decade. However, the issues confronting medical doctors went beyond pay and working conditions. Thatcher saw consensus-based policy-making as ineffective and sought to introduce sweeping reforms without relying on the corporatist approach (Greener, 2009). At the Conservative Party Conference in 1980, she made it clear that her set of policies was not up for discussion: 'You turn if you want to. The lady's not for turning' (Thatcher, 1980).

After the unrest of the 1970s, the medical profession's mobilisation was seen more as an attempt to trigger opposition than as an opportunity to develop support for change (Klein, 2013). In contrast with the principle underpinning the 1948 concordat, the medical profession was perceived less as a negotiating partner and more as an actor with vested interests.

The Thatcher government moved away from using ad hoc Committees and Royal Commissions to produce consensual proposals for reform. In 1983, Thatcher brought in an external figure from the business sector, Roy Griffiths, to look at ways to radically change organisational dynamics in the NHS.

Griffiths identified doctors as the natural managers of the service, which obviously earned the approval of the medical profession. But the government ignored this part of his advice and transferred managerial responsibilities from doctors to career administrators. The medical profession was not given an opportunity to discuss these changes, and had to accept them as a *fait accompli*.

Professional autonomy was further challenged by a reform to limit the range of drug prescriptions that could be made by a GP. The proposal emerged from a 1984 review, once again instigated by the government without participation from the medical profession. Unsurprisingly, the BMA, as well as the RCGP and GMSC, objected, with GPs striking an unlikely alliance with pharmaceutical companies and the Labour opposition party to protest the Bill.

This episode revealed fragmentation in the medical profession, with the Royal Colleges coming out in favour of the change. GPs obtained some concessions but, in a further sign of the government's willingness to push through despite medical opposition, the reform was introduced in February 1985.

GPs had a further confrontation with the government over the renewal of their contract. The government's proposals, including new incentive payments, were not particularly controversial in and of themselves, but the BMA still displayed irritation (General Medical Services Committee, 1986). This contrasted with the *BMJ*'s more conciliatory tone as it highlighted some of the positive aspects of the financial incentives (*BMJ*, 1986).

Publication of the 1989 plan *Working for Patients* turned the long negotiations into a full-blown confrontation when the medical profession became upset about government modifications to previously agreed positions. The heated exchanges were fairly predictable, but a last-minute rejection of the agreement by rank-and-file GPs was unexpected. It revealed a lack of faith in their negotiators. However, GPs did not see fit to take job action, and Health Secretary Clarke took advantage of the collective hesitation in the medical profession to push through the new GP contract in April 1990.

The medical profession was again excluded from the 1988 review of the NHS, which was conducted by a small team of senior ministers, chaired by Prime Minister Thatcher and supported by civil servants and political advisers (Timmins, 1995). Taking a page from Bevan's playbook, Clarke refused to engage in conversations with the leaders of the profession and instead sought advice from a few like-minded individuals (Greener, 2009).

In an open challenge to medical doctors' autonomy, the resulting White Paper of 1989 imposed greater accountability, with managers (at least in theory) being given the power to assess doctors' performance, oversee pay awards and decide disciplinary matters. Despite opposition from the medical profession and patient organisations, these plans were passed into law in 1990, testifying to the sheer determination of Health Secretary Clarke.

As in 1948, the medical profession harboured resentment not just about the content of the reform, but also about the government's policy-making approach. Some elements of the reform – including GP fundholding – were adopted even without prior warning to the BMA. In the main, GPs appreciated that they were made responsible for resource management, including hospital services: 'I [a GP fundholder] thought this is a revolution happening here. No consultant has ever talked to me about what I might think of his service, or any of the general problems we might have in twenty years of professional life' (cited in Rivett, 1998: 425). However, the government's radicalism in pushing the changes through Parliament without consultation or concessions enraged the medical profession.

The introduction of a system of performance indicators proved less contentious. Despite reassurance, since the creation of the NHS, that medical doctors would remain free from outside intervention in clinical or practice matters, even doctors appreciated that they needed to be more transparent about their daily practices (*BMJ*, 1980). The introduction of performance indicators raised the possibility that acceptable standards of performance, although set by the medical profession, could eventually be questioned and contribute to eroding professional autonomy.

Implications for medical politics and healthcare reforms

This period of reforms represented a clear break from the previous policy-making style characterised by bargaining between the government and the medical profession (Ham, 2009). Policy shifts became more sudden and the government was not afraid of provoking strong opposition.

The government's disregard extended to medical unions, which, in contrast to the driving force they represented in the 1970s, were relegated to being rather passive spectators in the 1980s (Klein, 2013). Thatcher and Clarke repeatedly demonstrated their resolve to face down the medical profession, unafraid of the potential impact on their own popularity or on GPs' acrimony.

The first significant reform of the 1980s – the imposition of general managers – caught the medical profession off guard. They were shocked by the government's determination and lacked the ability to resist. The change represented a major challenge to medical doctors who had controlled NHS resources for the last 40 years.

Following Griffiths' recommendations, doctors were still involved in resource allocation, and became more accountable for their decisions. They also lost their veto power in management committees (Klein, 2013). The language of management became the reference point for discussions around resources (Bloomfield and Best, 1992). Thus, the conditions leading to the original 'concordat' changed, with the government acquiring a more prominent role in running the NHS.

The creation of the internal market in the NHS represented a further shift in the dynamics between the State and medical profession. Prior to 1989, the relationship between the two protagonists was anchored in trust and respect for the initial concordat, although there had been signs of fracture in this informal arrangement.

The medical profession became increasingly critical of government during the 1980s, and this went beyond traditional pay disputes. Resentment ran deeper and stemmed from the feeling that government efforts to solve the funding crisis posed more serious threats (Klein, 2013). The internal market questioned the principles underpinning medical practice, with the government seeming to think that financial incentives rather than professional ethical considerations would motivate doctors to behave differently (that is, more efficiently).

Labour in power: (re)engineered consensus, 1997–2010

The influence of context: drivers and shapers of medical politics

After nearly two decades of Conservative government, Labour's election victory presented an opportunity to return to a more conciliatory style of policy-making. The Blair government recognised the benefits of some of the reforms introduced during the Conservative years, and also sought to distance itself from 'old Labour's' approach to healthcare policy (Ham, 2009). Most significant in the government plan was renewed trust in primary care to serve as the driving force in the system by aligning 'clinical and financial responsibility' (Secretary of State for Health, 1997: 9).

Beyond organisational dynamics, the government was also keen to use a number of mechanisms to raise clinical standards, assuming that self-regulation by the medical profession was not capable of delivering the expected improvements. The medical profession could have perceived this as an adversarial move, but high-profile medical scandals made the existing arrangements untenable, and the GMC had to acquiesce. This period was also characterised by a bonanza in terms of resource availability, as strong economic conditions facilitated continued growth in annual NHS budgets.

When overall performance did not improve, as promised, the government rather impatiently launched *The NHS Plan* to achieve 'a health service designed around the patient' (Secretary of State for Health, 2000: 10). Looking back at this reform, Prime Minister Blair recalled: 'the idea was then, over time, to move to a radically different type of service, abandoning the old monolithic NHS and replacing it with one devolved and decentralised with far greater power in the hands of the patient' (quoted in Rivett, 1998). Control over much of the NHS' overall budget was given to a new form of commissioning organisation –PCTs – again emphasising reliance on the market-type approach of previous Conservative governments (DH, 2001).

As a further vote of confidence in the positive effects of competitive pressures, high performing Hospital Trusts were given the opportunity to become more independent and retain any surplus they generated by transforming into Foundation Trusts. This policy was criticised by some Labour Party members as well as trade unions, seeing it as a dangerous move towards privatisation of the NHS (Shaw, 2007); the medical profession silently approved. NHS staff had repeatedly denounced excessive centralisation and micro-management, so devolution of control to the local level was favourably received.

Another measure that appeared uncharacteristic for a Labour government was to give the private sector greater opportunity to run diagnostic and treatment centres in order to reduce wait times. Once more, the medical profession saw little need to object, despite the similarity with reform ideas that underpinned the internal market of the Conservative period – and had, at the time, provoked serious confrontations with medical doctors.

The Labour period concluded with Prime Minister Gordon Brown instructing, in July 2007, a prominent clinician, Lord Ara Darzi, to conduct a wide-ranging review to plan the next set of reforms. The final report, *High Quality Care for All* (Secretary of State for Health,

2008), highlighted the urgent need to improve the quality of healthcare and patient safety and increase staff engagement in leadership roles to drive improvement.

This was in every respect a proposal formulated and led by the medical profession. Among other things, it advocated restoring to clinicians the responsibility for leading and managing healthcare organisations. The report was a landmark document that spearheaded crucial changes in the education and training of aspiring doctors.

Strategies used by the protagonists to accommodate and deal with the evolving context

The Labour period was marked by the medical profession's more supportive and constructive stance. The BMA greeted the 1997 White Paper positively, even if some of the measures represented a threat to the traditional autonomy of the profession. This was due in part to a sense of vindication – the reasons for its opposition to the Thatcher reforms were explicitly recognised as legitimate by the Labour government – and in part because some of the issues that proved problematic only emerged during the implementation phase (Klein, 2013). In return for meaningful support for the reform programme, the government promised more significant investment, including new contracts for GPs and specialists.

However, it was the Blair government's approach to health policy-making that deserved most credit for the amicable relationship with the medical profession during this period. This was exemplified by the use of collaborative policy tools such the Modernisation Action Teams that were instructed, in 2000, to work on *The NHS Plan*.

The medical profession was enthusiastically engaged with the formulation of the White Paper, perhaps even energised by the struggles and exclusion it had faced during the Conservative period. Of the more than 100 changes discussed, the BMA only objected to one that would impede early career specialists from exercising in private practice.

The BMA was also reassured by government recognition that more resources were needed in the NHS, including additional staff. The government's aim of achieving consensus by mobilising doctors came to fruition, with the *BMJ* suggesting that this was 'as good as it gets' (Dixon and Dewar, 2000).

Similarly, GPs had no objection to the government's renewed focus on GPs' leadership role in the NHS. They had accepted GP fundholding in the 1990s, and did not oppose the Labour reforms meant to enable greater patient choice (Greener, 2009). In a sense, the Labour policy was based on the same principles as the 1989 White Paper *Working for Patients* that gave GPs a more central role in the provision of care.

More ground breaking was the shift in primary care provision generated by the new GP contract that introduced, alongside the traditional GMS contract, a PMS option. This meant adopting the principle of flexible salaried employment for GPs, who had, since the inception of the NHS, operated as self-employed private contractors.

Particularly significant was the decision by Health Secretary Alan Milburn to transfer responsibility for contract negotiations to an inexperienced body, the NHS Confederation, at the first sign of disagreement from the medical profession. This turned out to be a costly decision for the government as the inexperienced negotiators could not withstand the full 'assault' by the medical profession; according to one policy-maker: 'the Department [of Health] was shafted' (cited in Klein, 2013: 237).

A more contentious pattern was observed during the specialist contract negotiations. The government and specialists agreed that the existing contract needed substantial updating, but did not see eye to eye as far as private practice was concerned. Labour had signalled its intention to reduce pay beds back in the 1970s, but the BMA was particularly opposed to the idea of curtailing specialists' ability to practise outside the NHS.

Negotiations lasted two years until, in June 2002, the government conceded to some of the requests and awarded pay increases in return for a modest increase in control over specialists. As happened repeatedly in the history of the NHS, doctors rejected the proposal despite it being supported by the BMA, leading to the resignation of the main negotiator, BMA Central Consultants and Specialists Committee Chair, Dr Peter Hawker. The contract was only approved after some of the government's accountability demands were softened.

Beyond the customary skirmishes around compensation, the medical profession attracted intense scrutiny from the government and the public due to a series of tragic events including the Bristol Royal Infirmary scandal (where numerous babies died after heart surgery), and the murder of over 200 patients by Dr Harold Shipman. Inquiries into these events were sobering to the medical profession, which recognised that maintaining the status quo was not an option.

The *BMJ* discussed the shortcomings of GMC regulation, and admitted that the issues at the Bristol Royal Infirmary were not exclusive to this hospital (Dyer, 2001). Indeed, the Kennedy Inquiry (2001) concluded that 'the most essential tool in achieving, sustaining, and improving quality of care for the patient was lacking ... clinicians had to satisfy only themselves that the service was of sufficient quality'.

Evidence presented at the Shipman Inquiry (Smith, 2002) put the final nail in the coffin for the existing system of professional self-regulation, noting 'fundamental flaws' associated with the role of the GMC. The Inquiry lead, Dame Janet Smith, stated that 'the leopard [the GMC] had not changed its spots' after the Bristol scandal (Smith, 2004). The GMC was directly in the line of fire, with even the *BMJ* claiming that it was time for radical reform (Kmietowicz, 2005).

A modified form of self-regulation was maintained, but at the cost of increased accountability and more limited autonomy at the individual level (Klein, 2013). Medical malpractice and negligence were once and for all placed outside the exclusive control of the medical profession, in particular the Royal Colleges and the GMC.

Implications for medical politics and healthcare reforms

In stark contrast with the Conservative period, the Labour era was characterised by the government's willingness to keep professionals on their side. The medical profession found it relatively unproblematic to negotiate rewarding pay settlements. Nevertheless, this period also witnessed a substantial erosion of professional autonomy in terms of self-regulation, accountability and performance standards.

Furthermore, the Labour government's openness to authorising additional roles for alternative providers implied that one of the two pillars of the 'double bed' relationship was crumbling. The State was, to an extent, becoming less reliant on keeping the medical profession content working in the public sector. The relationship between the protagonists began to shift from structurally necessary to contingency dependent (Greener, 2009).

This process had begun under the Conservative governments of the 1980s, but Labour gave it a new lease on life. Conservative Health Secretary Clarke adopted an adversarial approach with the medical profession, introducing health reforms without directly consulting doctors, and even openly opposing their views.

In contrast, Labour's stance was more conciliatory, although this did not mean that the government would refrain from pushing the boundaries of what might be acceptable to the medical profession. Medical doctors appeared less inclined to resort to active resistance and confrontation, perhaps because pay settlements were particularly generous during this period.

Building on the notion of managerialism introduced by the Conservatives under Thatcher, the Labour period also brought enhanced scrutiny and regulation of the medical profession. The government became more forceful in its dealings with doctors, demanding greater accountability at the individual level as well as in relation to their professional bodies.

The introduction of organisations such as NICE challenged the assumptions underlying traditional medical practice. Clinical priorities had to be balanced against the financial implications of a treatment, which needed to be clinically cost-effective (Greener, 2009). The development of clinical governance then exposed hospital doctors, and particularly specialists, to an unprecedented level of scrutiny. Doctors became more accountable within their organisations, and their decisions and actions were closely examined by managers. Accountability to peers was supplemented by accountability to employers.

Management in the NHS increasingly became a local responsibility, and both the GMC and employers exercised control over medical practice. At the same time, managerialism in policy-making, initially despised but gradually, and at times grudgingly, accepted, led the medical profession to take an increasingly tough stance as the defender of patient care and the public character of the NHS against the budget-driven demands of the state.

The coalition period and a return to conflict, 2010–20

The influence of context: drivers and shapers of medical politics

The outcome of the 2010 General Election seemed to signal a period of relative calm in the NHS. The first priority of the new coalition government was to agree on a common strategy to support economic recovery after the global financial crisis of 2007/08. The political class and society more generally were caught off guard, therefore, when the new Secretary of State for Health, Andrew Lansley, released the White Paper *Equity and Excellence: Liberating the NHS* in July 2010.

The policy paper included radical reforms that rivalled the 1989 *Working for Patients* plan. The proposals included – not for the first time in the NHS – devolving power and putting front-line clinicians in the driver's seat. Some ideas corresponded to the 2008 Darzi report, but the extent of the planned structural reorganisation of the NHS was, according to Chief Executive Sir David Nicholson, unquestionably 'revolutionary'.

Rather surprisingly for a conservative politician, Lansley believed that, to be successful, changes in the NHS would have to be led bottom-up by the medical profession. Whether or not the profession was willing to take on this role did not seem to concern the Health Secretary. In a remarkable shift of power and accountability, GPs were required to assume, almost overnight, the leading role in commissioning (Timmins, 2012). This raised significant concern across the medical profession.

The next Secretary of State for Health, Jeremy Hunt, also antagonised the medical profession, attempting, soon after a majority Conservative government took power in 2015, to impose drastic changes to the contract with junior doctors. The resulting hostility between the government and the medical profession on this issue was so acute that it took almost three years from the time the contract was unilaterally imposed to reach a compromise.

In terms of significant health reforms, there was little activity in the NHS in the years following the acrimonious events linked to Lansley's 2012 Health and Social Care Act (Health and Social Care Act, 2012). This was partly attributable to the emergence of other important political events (notably the 2016 Brexit Referendum) but also to the approach adopted by the Chief Executive of NHS England, Simon Stevens.

In the 2014 5YFV, Stevens attempted to build on existing service developments, essentially aiming to achieve 're-organisation without reform' (Exworthy et al, 2016). Prioritising the integration of health and social care provision, this strategy sought to facilitate a bottom-up approach by working in partnership with the medical profession away from direct political involvement. The outcomes of this approach are, at the time of this writing, still difficult to see, especially with the number of factors contributing to slow down progress.

Strategies used by the protagonists to accommodate and deal with the evolving context

Lansley wanted to introduce a programme of reforms that would outlast future political interventions. The scope and scale of his ambitious programme were aimed for the long term, with the goal of introducing a definitive solution to problems that had affected the NHS up to that point. He chose to reveal little about the plans, including to his own political party, and their implications were fully understood only when the White Paper was translated into a parliamentary Bill.

Once again, the medical profession's reaction was mixed. Not unexpectedly, the BMA's GP committee had a favourable view of GP commissioning (Timmins, 2012), while the rest of the BMA reacted negatively to the proposed reforms. Criticism drew on well-oiled arguments used against the Thatcher reforms, including 'that increased commercialisation has not been beneficial for the NHS or the patients' (BMA, 2010).

In alignment with the RCGP, the BMA had long supported 'an NHS untarnished by a market economy' (Timmins, 2008), to avoid big business 'taking money out of the NHS' and placing 'profits before patients' (Timmins, 2010). Tellingly, both representative bodies sustained their opposition despite the plethora of amendments made to the Bill in Parliament.

The other Royal Colleges were less forthcoming than the BMA in rejecting the proposals, but still maintained a 'critical engagement' with Lansley's plans (Klein, 2013). At the other end of the spectrum, niche associations – NHS Alliance and the National Association of Primary Care – representing groups of GPs perceived the plan as an opportunity to achieve 'emancipation'.

The main concern of many GPs and the BMA was the double-edged sword that giving GPs direct control over commissioning represented. It meant more freedom and influence over decision-making at the local level, but also further raised the bar on accountability. In the plan, GPs were expected to simultaneously act in the interest of patients and as 'agents of the State' responsible for how public money was spent, that is, for rationing resources. According to Dr Clare Gerada, Council Chair of the RCGP, making GPs 'the new rationalisers' would certainly cause irreparable damage to the doctor–patient relationship (Campbell, 2010).

Although Lansley loathed to retreat from his plans, the sheer scale of criticism forced the coalition government to announce an unprecedented 'pause' for reflection and consultation, in particular with the medical profession. The reforms had become the government's 'biggest domestic political headache' and, sensing an opportunity, the BMA kept up its opposition to the Bill (Timmins, 2012).

The government attempted to bring doctors on board by giving them control over changes in the proposed reforms. The ad hoc NHS Future Forum provided the conduit for the medical profession's expression of agency. It was chaired by an expert in primary care, Professor Steve Field, and doctors made up a third of its members.

The Future Forum report was published within two months and the government wasted no time in accepting most of its recommendations. The medical profession managed to put its definitive stamp on the legislation, with the Royal Colleges and grassroots doctors' associations insisting on several further amendments during parliamentary debate.

A similar pattern of exchanges characterised negotiations (or the lack thereof) for the junior doctors' contract. The Health Secretary was determined to end dangerous working patterns for junior doctors, whom he saw as overworked and insufficiently supported by more experienced doctors, especially at weekends. Doctors, on the other hand, saw his proposals as an attempt to save on overtime costs and relentlessly opposed – at some points against the advice of their professional representatives – any agreement that would compromise their compensation.

Rather uniquely in the history of the NHS, Health Secretary Hunt unilaterally imposed the new contract on junior doctors when negotiations failed to produce results. The confrontation that followed between the government and the medical profession reached unprecedented levels, with junior doctors repeatedly striking and bringing legal cases to court.

Implications for medical politics and healthcare reforms

The outcome of Lansley's reform was that the government had to retreat and revise its proposals in the face of concerted opposition from the medical profession. More than 2,000 amendments were made to the original plan during parliamentary debate. Although doctors did not form a fully united front, they were the driving force in discussions and ensured that changes were made in line with their professional interests.

This provided further evidence that the medical profession had come a long way from the Conservative period of the 1980s–90s, when it had been marginalised (or ostracised) in the policy-making process. Unlike the Thatcher government reforms, which were enshrined in law despite the objections of the medical profession, the government's response during the Lansley plan debate reaffirmed the power of the medical profession to shape health policy, power that Conservative governments had openly questioned and sometimes even tamed. The coalition government, perhaps in part because it was internally split along different party objectives, lacked the will to impose reforms on the medical profession.

A parallel observation can be made in relation to the fraught negotiations over the junior doctors' contract. The Health Secretary wanted to maintain a hard line in what he saw as a necessary change in working patterns, but the sheer force and resolve of the medical profession's opposition eventually led him to retreat.

Never before in the history of the NHS had a contract been imposed on doctors, and they refused to be shoved into a contractual arrangement they perceived as punitive. The eventual modification of the contract with terms more agreeable to the medical profession once again demonstrated that doctors would not be easily subjugated to changes that went against their interests.

5

Comparative analysis

In this section, we present a set of analytical themes and considerations derived from our analysis of the three empirical cases in England and Canada. The intent is to elucidate the implications of our research on how we understand the medical doctor–healthcare reform nexus and to test our theoretical model's ability to explain key variations and points of convergence across the cases.

We first examine the impact on healthcare reforms of the deals and policy parameters set at the inception of PFHS. We identify foundational elements that set the scene for future debates and negotiations between the government and medical doctors in the development of reforms. Contextual factors push governments into this most significant health reform, and the creation of PFHS is a revelatory moment. It shows how the two protagonists become engaged in a common endeavour with different expectations and abilities to influence the architecture of the system. The spirit of the initial agreement and the growing interdependence between governments and the medical profession has enduring implications for their future relationship.

Second, we delineate how governments address core policy dilemmas in the context of PFHS. Manifestations of the agency of governments within the mediated space of reforms are shaped by intense political pressures to respond to dilemmas such as escalating costs and problems with access to care. They also interface with the medical profession's reactions to reformative propositions. On the one hand, governments need to secure the collaboration of a powerful insider, the medical profession, and mobilise a diversity of policy instruments that go beyond coercion. On the other hand, the medical profession's contestation of propositions, and the limited ability for protagonists to genuinely engage in large-scale joint policy-making, creates situations where governments attempt to impose – usually minor – policy changes through coercion.

Third, we characterise the institution of medical politics as a core feature of contemporary PFHS that operates as a determining influence on healthcare reforms. While governments learn through their policy work the challenges of reforming PFHS and securing the support of medical doctors, the medical profession builds its political clout on the experience of exchanges with governments. Getting involved in health reforms is a significant political experience for the medical profession. It also reveals a specific representation by the medical profession of its own position within

PFHS and of governments' legitimate role. The institution of medical politics consolidates over time and becomes an inherent feature of the medical profession. It incorporates a political credo that significantly influences manifestations of the medical profession's agency within the mediated space of reforms.

Fourth, we focus on the interface of agentic manifestations by medical doctors and governments in the mediated space to identify their influence on the evolution of each other's respective strategies. While contextual forces are often catalysts for reforms, the two protagonists develop various approaches to influence each other within the mediated space. Governments oscillate between collaborative and coercive approaches when seeking the support of the medical profession. Decisions about approaches to policy-making are influenced by the reactions of the medical profession and the intensity of pressures from the distal and proximal context. Governments clearly appear as the initiator of reforms and generate momentum within the mediated space. The medical profession is more reactive and engages within that space as a receiver of changes. The medical profession is an active claimant around aspects related to status and working conditions, but plays a less generative role in broader health policy issues. Predispositions to change, as revealed by the political credo associated with medical politics, significantly shape the medical profession's determination to meaningfully engage in reforms.

Fifth, we assess how configurations of these four dimensions of the medical doctor–healthcare reform nexus influence the content of reformative templates over time. To various degrees, the comparative analysis reveals that the relationship between the medical profession and the PFHS limits prospects for reform. For the most part, predispositions to change and the political practices that have developed in the mediated space of reforms limit the scope for change.

There are, however, some variations across our empirical cases and situations where the medical profession engages in broader health policy issues. Based on our empirical findings, we can identify pathways for change that shape compliance with and/or the reframing of proposed reforms.

Setting the scene: the political meanings of inception

Historical accounts of the founding moments and evolving trajectories of PFHS in various jurisdictions, including for England and Canada, abound in the literature (Webster, 1988; Maioni, 1997; Tuohy, 1999; Ham, 2009; Klein, 2013). The first objective of our analysis was to focus on these foundational moments as revelatory antecedents of the predispositions of our two protagonists. We concentrated on the specific manifestations of their agency within the mediated space that impact on the adoption of a policy framework in support of a PFHS. Policy frameworks established at the outset of the system were considered critical elements in setting the stage for further exchanges between governments and the medical profession (Webster, 1988; Klein, 2013; Lazar et al, 2013; Baggott, 2015; Tuohy, 2018). The inception of the PFHS was the result of a cluster of political forces and contextual factors (distal and proximal) that created policy momentum in favour of significant policy change. In both countries, policy activism was evident years before the adoption of acts creating the PFHS.

In the negotiations that precede the creation of the PFHS, we observed in all three cases policy compromise around the mutual obligations and expectations of the medical profession and governments. Debates around the emergence of the PFHS revealed the values and interests put forward by and explicitly confronted by the two protagonists. During this period, governments (the Westminster government in England and the federal government in Canada) pursued a clear expansion of the state's welfare agenda (Maioni, 2004; Klein, 2013). The experience of the Second World War – more acute in the case of England – coupled with post-war economic growth provided governments with the legitimacy to think about and implement progressive social policies. The UK Labour government embarked on a vast programme of nationalisation, and the health service formed a key piece of that puzzle, particularly after the Beveridge report (1942). Furthermore, like other European countries, the UK experienced the inadequacy of the hospital care provision during the Second World War and the effectiveness of coordinated emergency services. Canada had to meet the healthcare needs of soldiers coming back from war. Universal access to care was at the top of the policy agenda in both countries, with governments recognising its importance for the general population and anticipating important developments in medicine. There was therefore a clear political advantage to moving forward with the idea of a PFHS.

The medical profession in the three cases was conscious that this meant embarking on a decisive adventure where government's expanding role and increasing control in health affairs would confront the values, interests and aspirations of medical doctors in various ways. The level of integration of the medical profession within the newly established systems reflected the tensions between governments and the profession. Our cases revealed clear variations with regard to the manifestation of such confrontations.

In England, the government was tenacious in pushing its policy agenda, while making some compromises. It maintained the self-employed status of GPs, but significantly changed the positions of medical doctors within the system by making hospital specialists employees of the NHS. While policy exchanges were not all cordial, and were at times lengthy and rather transactional, the medical profession ended up coming on board to create a universal system of care in 1948, two years after the enactment of the foundational Act (NHS Act 1946). The medical profession responded positively to contextual factors, pressure from the general population and a united political spectrum to cooperate in an important policy shift.

In Canada, in the early 1960s, the Canadian Medical Association (CMA) opposed the creation of a PFHS. Within the two sub-national jurisdictions explored in the cases, the medical profession as a whole displayed resistance and ambivalence. In Ontario, government intrusion in health affairs was met with suspicion from the outset. The medical profession actively promoted an improved health insurance programme to cover the costs of care for the less affluent. It saw this option as a guarantee of professional autonomy and self-regulation. In Québec, the medical profession did not voice policy alternatives as explicitly as in Ontario. GPs, perceived as second-class medical practitioners, were willing to participate in negotiations that would improve their status and economic situation. Specialist doctors were more reluctant, demanding regulations to protect the voluntary nature of adherence to the nascent PFHS. As in England, strong support from the population encouraged the government in Québec to move ahead, imposing rules to encourage the participation of medical doctors in the new system. Opting out became financially unattractive, which ensured the integration of the medical profession in the system.

In all three cases, the medical profession was assimilated into the new system, but its adherence and commitment varied and were notably stronger in England. This was likely associated with the government's decision to initially give medical professionals full control to operate medical services in the NHS without direct state intervention. But in all three cases, the fear of being under the government's control challenged the ethos of the medical profession. In Canada, a fundamental element of the new PFHS was the medical profession becoming an endogenous force animated by scepticism regarding the role of government in healthcare.

In England, the creation of the NHS came with an understanding that medical doctors would relinquish some of their bargaining power to the State. Having established a national system financed through general taxation, doctors would rely mainly on political pressure for leverage in future negotiations (Fredman and Morris, 1989). The State also had a firm upper hand as it gave itself full discretion in approving the terms and conditions of medical doctors' employment through the power vested in the Minister of Health (Secretary of State for Health) (Part I, section 1, NHS Act 1946).

The policy momentum around the creation of the PFHS also tested whether the political apparatus of the medical profession was sufficiently robust to navigate the new policy landscape. Within the mediated space activated around the PFHS, the medical profession in Québec felt the need for a robust political machine to voice values, principles, interests, demands and aspirations. With the recognition in the mid-1960s of three medical unions (the FMOQ, FMSQ and FMRQ), consolidation was relatively straightforward, and unions became emblematic of organised medicine. Political consolidation went hand in hand with the institutionalisation of separate political channels for GPs and specialists. In Ontario, the political machine was more fragmented, with persistent wavering around who represented the profession, and whether representative associations should have a monopoly in negotiations with government. Despite the fact that GPs and specialists were united in a single association, the OMA, the medical profession hesitated about delegating it monopoly representational power. This was in line with the medical profession's reluctance to participate in a PFHS and attachment to some form of health insurance market. In England, a fragmented polity, based partly on the BMA and the Royal Colleges of Medicine sharing duties of representation, did not create fertile ground for a unified approach to voicing the aspirations of the medical profession. The political division between specialists and GPs was institutionalised within the design of the new PFHS. Not represented by the Royal Colleges and unsatisfied with negotiations conducted by the BMA on their behalf, GPs refused to accept government demands long after hospital specialists adhered to the creation of a PFHS.

During the inception period, both protagonists repositioned themselves within a new context that forced them to openly state their values, interests and aspirations. In general terms, the creation of the PFHS integrated within the public sphere the management of the fundamental relationship in healthcare, namely, the relationship between the State as sole payer and the medical profession. It institutionalised the medical profession and the State as the main decision-makers in the health policy sphere (Tuohy, 2018). While recognising that the debates that preceded the creation of the PFHS were privileged windows on the positions and predispositions of the two protagonists, the extent to which this foundational bargain persisted and impacted health policy and reforms through time was surprising (Klein, 2013; Lazar et al, 2013; Tuohy, 2018). The creation of the PFHS in the three cases set the stage, the tone and the boundaries for further policy debates and exchanges between the medical profession and government. The medical profession became *de facto* a public profession, as its survival hinged on its relationship with the State (Ackroyd et al, 1989; Ackroyd, 2016), and this, despite its capacity to defend professional autonomy and self-regulation. It remained an influential decision-maker and insider in the new PFHS (Lazar et al, 2013). Both protagonists 'share the same bed' (Klein, 2013) and their interdependencies nurtured a logic of accommodation in the making of health policy. Accommodation did not always translate into policy consensus, but institutionalised inherent tensions between the State and the profession, including around hierarchy and peer control within the new system (Tuohy, 2018). Accordingly, governments became regulators as well as overseeing the system, and exerted pressure to strike a balance between different and potentially competing interests and imperatives, while also engaging some accommodation practices. The ability of governments to succeed in this challenging policy landscape constitutes one of the main empirical questions of our comparative analysis.

Manifestations of the agency of the medical profession were mostly iterative and practical-evaluative (Emirbayer and Mishe, 1998) as the proposition of creating a PFHS confronted an ingrained representation of medical professionalism privileging professional autonomy and self-regulation, and the risks and opportunities associated with the new system. However, in Ontario and England, alternative propositions for an improved insurance market were put forward, demonstrating the medical profession's willingness to project itself into the future. Whether this was fundamentally an attempt to maintain the status quo or a concerted intention to assume a more progressive role in the health system remained questionable. In all three cases, the medical profession ultimately signed on and, most strikingly in Canada, was able to foresee and rapidly enjoy the advantages of being an independent entrepreneur without financial risks and benefiting from the generosity of the public purse. In England, the medical profession's strong commitment to the values of a PFHS was much more tangible. Although governments felt that proposing such a transformative health policy agenda was legitimate at the time, in Ontario, the government was more hesitant as it faced strong lobbying from the insurance sector. In Québec, strong support from the population and GPs for the creation of a PFHS provided important political traction for government to proceed with reforms despite opposition (from the insurance sector and specialists). The creation of the PFHS in all three cases was a remarkable achievement in scope and scale. The encounters between the two protagonists in the period around the inception of these systems strongly influenced how the two would debate, confront one another and reach agreement in the future. These exchanges also impacted how medical politics were structured, including differences in the segmentation of the medical profession (GPs and hospital specialists, for example) and in the roles of professional associations or unions in representing medical interests.

The initial agreements underpinned the organic relationship between the State and the medical profession. In this policy context, the logic of accommodation appeared a natural outcome of the institutionalisation of medical politics within the politics of welfare states (Tuohy, 2018). Exogenous and endogenous forces, including external shocks, introduced nuances or changes further down the road to the initial momentum observed within this dyadic relationship. In the three cases, exogenous forces put governments in a position to move forward with the creation of a PFHS, but with variable degrees of compromise with the medical profession. It was interesting to note how founding moments and experiences had an enduring impact on the making of health policies and reforms.

Manifestations of government agency: ruling in a conundrum

The creation of PFHS significantly increased and transformed the roles and responsibilities of governments in health affairs. While a significant role for government in health matters was not the prerogative of PFHS (see, for example, Starr, 1982; Quadagno, 2005; Patel and Rushefsky, 2014), the creation of a PFHS expanded the role of government as main decision-maker regarding the regulation and funding of healthcare. In the context of our study, the creation of PFHS put health policies at the top of the agenda in the emerging welfare states of England and Canada. The specificities of health policies, with their ambition to ensure maximum coverage for all, their growing costs linked to medical discoveries, and the singular status of the medical profession, generated important policy dilemmas that were faced by governments across our period of study (Forest and Denis, 2012). As noted previously, while exchanges between the medical profession and governments pre-dated the creation of PFHS, these systems made the medical profession a crucial insider. In their role as regulators and financing entities, governments in all three cases interacted significantly with the medical profession inside the mediated space. Medical politics were not a feature unique to PFHS, as exemplified by the key role played by the medical profession in health policy in the US (Laugesen, 2016). However, the PFHS provided a unique context of interdependency between government and the medical profession, increasing the odds of both intense activity and inertia in the policy arena.

In the Introduction, we defined government as an amalgamated set of institutions and authority that rely on diverse strategies to implement decisions and conceive innovative policies such as reforms (Robertson, 2002; Jensen, 2008; Jessop, 2011). The fundamental role played by institutions, such as governments, in the stabilisation or rebalancing of relationships among actors endowed with strong agentic capacities has been identified as one of the features of modern society (Meyer, 2010). By extension, one might argue that reforms are an opportunity to address and rebalance the relationship between the institution of government and the institution of the medical profession (Leicht, 2005; Leicht and Fennell, 2008; Scott, 2008; Suddaby and Muzio, 2015). Governments rely on their agentic capacities to address the challenge of rebalancing their relationship with medical doctors in order to solve emerging policy dilemmas. The functioning of PFHS in the decades following their creation presented governments with numerous and complex policy dilemmas. For instance, governments had to find a balance, at times precarious, between cost and access to high quality care (Maynard, 2013). These policy dilemmas meant that the availability of resources, the state of public finances and other competing policy priorities conflicted, with different degrees of intensity, with the pre-dispositions and expectations of the medical profession. Empirically, many instances of policy conflict arose in the three cases, and were more acute in the two Canadian cases. In accomplishing this mandate, governments relied on a variety of policy instruments to frame exchanges with the medical profession, communicate governments' imperatives and jointly find solutions (Schneider and Ingram, 1990; Lascoumes and Le Galès, 2007).

Tuohy (2018) has described government reforms as generally structured around a policy framework that determines how various groups will interact within a given policy sector, which policy instruments will mediate their interactions and how actors are held accountable for their decisions and behaviour. Within our three cases, governments proposed reformative ideas on a cyclical basis and acted as first port of call when stakeholders, including the medical profession, voiced concerns regarding the functioning and performance of the health system. We compared how governments chose to inhabit the mediated space around the medical profession and the State, what imperatives or strategic intentions they engaged in the space, and how they mobilised policy instruments to exert influence.

The way the English government fulfilled its role as a reformer and decision-maker in the health system contrasted with the roles assumed by Québec and Ontario governments in Canada. Over more than 70 years, Westminster actively proposed policy changes, despite having entered the mediated space more discretely during the first 30 years of the NHS. Indeed, although the English government was conscious of growing healthcare costs, problems with the governance and maintenance of healthcare facilities, and medical professionals' discontent with compensation levels, for nearly three decades it maintained a collaborative relationship with the medical profession, marred by only sporadic and fairly minimal tensions. The fragmented polity within the profession may have helped create and sustain this concordat. On the one hand, specialists had access to the political elite and could more directly express their views, preoccupations and demands. GPs often had to enter into public conflicts with the government in order to promote and protect their interests. This established a more confrontational dynamic, where GPs used job action as a bargaining chip (for example, during negotiations in the 1960s that ultimately resulted in the Charter for the Family Doctor Service). Despite policy reports highlighting the need to improve GPs' working and financial conditions (for example, the 1960 report of the Royal Commission on Doctors' and Dentists' Remuneration), it took the concrete threat of a strike for government to respond to their demands.

To a certain extent, the government attempted to resolve systemic problems by entering the negotiated space with a collaborative approach to policy-making. Instances of joint policy-making with the medical profession characterised the relationship with specialists, as seen with the *Hospital Plan* of the 1960s. Policy instruments mobilised during this consensual period were mainly incentive tools (Schneider and Ingram, 1990) – such as increases in remuneration – capacity and learning tools, and policy reports. Events in subsequent periods suggested that the government was willing to play a more confrontational role with the medical profession. It was also willing to use its authority to impose changes, including an incentive scheme that promoted healthcare provider accountability and helped rationalise healthcare spending. Accordingly, the Conservative governments imposed a managerialist approach without consulting the medical profession or securing its support. The government also adopted a confrontational approach to introduce the internal market reforms spelled out in *Working for Patients* in 1989.

Subsequent reforms were characterised by greater collaboration and a return to the use of incentive and capacity building tools. After 1997, Labour governments made concerted efforts to highlight the role of the medical profession (symbolic tool) and the need to draw on its expertise in health reforms (learning tool). Reforms during that period thus relied on a greater diversity of policy instruments and favoured a more collaborative approach to interactions among healthcare organisations and providers, even while maintaining a market-oriented logic.

In the following decades, the coalition government and subsequent Conservative governments again displayed a willingness to impose major changes without extensive consultation with the profession in the mediated space. A push for consumerist reforms relying on a complex set of policy instruments to put GPs directly in charge of purchasing and rationing healthcare services led to another bitter confrontation between our two protagonists. The final version of the Act reflected the many changes made to the initial reformative proposals through the expert intervention of the medical profession.

In relation to the two Canadian cases, the first decade of the PFHS was relatively untroubled, with only a few episodes of conflict around medical compensation. However, the PFHS tested governments when they realised how much healthcare expenses and medical compensation were increasing. It became obvious that governments would have to pay greater attention to the demands and expectations of the medical profession, to what medical doctors offered the population in term of access to services, and to the profession's general views on the PFHS (see the next section on medical politics). Governments in Québec and Ontario entered the mediated space with growing constraints imposed by a formal regime of labour relations that became necessary to deal with health policy dilemmas – or at least with the medical profession.

Across all subsequent periods of reform, both governments (Ontario and Québec) faced greater challenges in their attempts to reconcile cost control and access to high-quality healthcare across their territories. Our detailed exploration of the consolidation and characteristics of the institution of medical politics showed that one of the key decision-makers, government, seemed to be relatively weak in promoting and materialising its reformative agenda. This was not because it was unable to mobilise a diverse set of policy instruments for reforms. As we saw in the Québec case, the government used sophisticated capacity and learning instruments such as public commissions to diagnose the state of the PFHS and identify policy options to reform the system. The Ontario government did this as well, although to a lesser extent (one major commission, reports by policy experts on various policy issues such as extra billing and primary care reforms). However, the ability to both generate reformative ideas and collaborate with the medical profession seemed, as in the Québec case, more limited. In both cases, this contrasted sharply with the government's capacity to use coercion and authority to rationalise and restructure the entire health system.

Overall, while the Québec and Ontario governments were able to drive rationalisation and restructuring, they were in a much weaker position when implementing a reformative agenda that directly touched on the status of medical doctors within the PFHS, their integration within the system and their compensation. That said, joint policy-making, in the form of learning and capacity tools, developed in the 1980s and 1990s in Québec to promote better allocation of medical doctors in the territory and integrate medical advice into the planning of medical labour within regional and central governance bodies. In Ontario, the medical profession participated in a joint policy-making committee with the Ontario government. Changes to the organisation of primary care in Québec and Ontario after 2000, and more specifically the reorganisation of private GP practices into family health teams or medical groups, were important policy moments that appeared, on the whole, to be both consensual and transformative. However, the cost of these reforms (see Marchildon and Hutchison, 2016 for the Ontario experience), and the difficulty of applying sophisticated and acceptable policy instruments to increase productivity, suggested that governments faced serious limits in playing the role of demanding payer and regulator of medical affairs. Joint policy-making became government's preferred option when it needed to transcend the limits of the labour relations regime, although it was not entirely sufficient to rebalance the government's relationship with the medical profession.

Overall, our analysis revealed that, to assert their reformative agenda, governments relied on a diverse set of policy instruments that evolved and changed across periods. The potential of these instruments to integrate medical doctors within the PFHS was particularly interesting. In Canada, most authoritative instruments (or threats to use them) seemed to lack efficiency in acting on immediate medical policy issues. More collaborative and learning instruments, that were in line with a predominant policy logic of accommodation, appeared more successful in bringing medical doctors on board around major policy dilemmas perceived by government. Nevertheless, at least in the Canadian cases, these instruments also limited governments' ability to promote, within the mediated space, transformative policies that directly impacted the medical profession. Reformative templates promoted by government constituted contestable narratives of governance (Bevir, 2010, 2013) and faced serious – and seemingly more intense in the Canadian cases – challenges from the medical profession. Progressively increasing challenges to government reforms were also noticeable in the English NHS. After the mid-1970s, a more chaotic relationship with the medical profession took hold, where the government consciously moved away from an accommodation strategy by favouring a more coercive and conflictual approach. As in the Canadian cases, however, the logic of accommodation re-emerged decisively when policies based on authoritative approaches required the medical profession to participate in their implementation. The reality of the mediated space implied that transformative policies would always be subject to the scrutiny and political intervention of the medical profession.

In all three cases, governments attempted to forge and promote new political rationalities to drive and govern the system, appealing to either a managerial credo of agility and modernisation, patient-centred care or democratic governance of the PFHS (Bevir, 2013; Martin and Waring, 2018). Changes in political rationalities embedded in reformative templates revealed a partial process of governmentalisation of the State, where governments aligned subjects only partially towards new political rationalities. In our three cases, governments' efforts in reforms seemed to have a limited impact on transforming the rationality that guided medical behaviours and practices. Our analysis of medical politics revealed the ideological substrate that guided involvement and resistance of the medical profession in reforms. The regulatory ambition of the State (Lodge, 2008) was highly visible across our three cases, while it failed to produce a new expression of medical professionalism within contemporary welfare states. Governments continued to diversify their policy instruments and tactics to find a way to reconcile their imperatives with the aspirations of the medical profession. They could act unilaterally through authoritative instruments, but the transformative impact of this approach appeared limited, at least in terms of forging and imposing a new regime of medical governmentality (see, for example, the Barrette reform in Québec or the internal market reforms in the English NHS). New rationalities and their associated governmental regimes were met with resistance in the Canadian cases (from both GPs and medical specialists to varying extents) and more tangible compliance from GPs in the context of NPM reforms in England, while also revealing political continuity in the position of medical doctors within the PFHS. The penetration of new logics varied across the Canadian and English cases. Governments' governmentality project, supported by its policy toolkit, was activated within a mediated space that had room for a certain amount of change, at least on the surface, but limited ability to bring about changes in mentality. Compliance with reforms mandated in the presence of a logic of accommodation did not, in the end, result in meaningful or significant transformations.

Manifestation of medical doctors' agency: medical politics as an institution in the making

The creation of PFHS initiated a long developmental or activation process of medical politics as a key institution within contemporary health policies. This process tended to amplify and formalise the political role of the medical profession in health affairs. Living the system from within and having governments as their main interlocutor, the medical profession embarked on a process of organising to strategically manage its relationship with a single payer and regulator. As an institution, medical politics appeared to be based on a complex set of values, norms and interests that aggregated in a more or less homogeneous political body. Thus, the notion of organised medicine captured this idea of a more formalised medical body and was associated with the development of formal channels to voice the medical profession's preferences regarding reformative agendas proposed by government.

Governments could not ignore the role and influence of medical politics in healthcare reforms in situations where the medical profession became an endogenous force and inside influencer in PFHS. Governments could even contribute to the structuration of medical politics in order to better navigate a frequently turbulent political landscape. Overall, in our cases, medical politics appeared as an institution in a state of becoming marked by the protagonists' experience of interactions in the mediated space associated with healthcare reforms. Medical politics were characterised by the more or less active (or generative) role of medical doctors in health reforms and policies. The evolution and manifestations of medical politics unfolded differently in the three empirical cases.

In our empirical findings, medical politics constituted a crucial institution for the evolution of contemporary PFHS – institution in the sense of 'more-or-less taken-for-granted repetitive social behaviour that is underpinned by normative systems and cognitive understandings that give meaning to social exchange and thus enable self-reproducing social order' (Greenwood et al, 2008: 4–5). As expressed in the exchanges between government and the medical profession within the mediated space, medical politics revealed repeating cognitive and normative patterns that influenced the perceptions of what it meant to be a medical doctor and of government's role in healthcare. Medical politics constituted a set of predispositions that influenced the way medical doctors, and consequently governments, deployed their agentic capacities. Through medical politics, the medical profession accomplished an institutional project that framed its relationship with PFHS (Suddaby and Viale, 2011). Across the three cases, medical politics influenced the way medical doctors conceived their own, and the government's, respective roles.

In the eyes of medical doctors, governments in the Canadian cases appeared as external intruders constantly attempting to transgress the foundational deal made with the medical profession at the creation of the PFHS as well as the essence of their profession. The medical profession became something akin to a public profession (despite mostly remaining private providers), and constantly had to deal with government's determination to renegotiate initial agreements (Ackroyd et al, 1989). In this context, a specific representation or interpretation of medical professionalism became institutionalised. From the perspective of the medical profession, the foundational deal involved a distant relationship between medical doctors and the PFHS. This view was associated with medical doctors' growing mistrust of government's regulatory ambitions. It fostered an ideological context in which medical doctors repeatedly expressed scepticism within the mediated space regarding the legitimate role of governments and bureaucrats and their added value.

Our data illustrated how governments' reformative initiatives were systematically perceived as attempts to corrupt an essentialist view of the medical profession. Medical doctors in Canada had an experience of the PFHS that was never totally normalised or tamed. Our analysis of discourses and exchanges within the mediated space by organised medicine revealed that medical doctors, and especially medical specialists, often felt like outcasts and outsiders of the system, and saw broader health policy issues as distractions. Thus, medical doctors' experience of the PFHS was, in very general terms, that of an *under-socialised* profession. This under-socialisation was nourished by an essentially backward-looking, iterative form of agency (Emirbayer and Mishe, 1998), in which the pre-PFHS period was represented mostly in idealised terms.

The ideological (cognitive and normative) substrate of medical politics revealed in the Canadian cases may be exaggerated in the sense that it did not capture some of the more collaborative expressions of medical politics. First, at least for the Québec case, GPs were more inclined, despite their own scepticism regarding governments and bureaucrats, to compromise and adhere to innovative policy ideas. Consequently, joint policy-making and involvement in policy roles sporadically emerged. The union of medical specialists (FMSQ) was more radical and reluctant to engage, and tended to systematically oppose reformative ideas promoted by government. It saw reforms as ineffective solutions to real-life problems, and perceived them as projects driven by bureaucratic rationalisers. The political credo of GPs and medical specialists shared common underpinnings; however, they differed in their level of adherence to this political view, their perceptions of reforms and their behaviour (through their unions) within the mediated space.

The Ontario case featured a more complex architecture of medical politics where, despite GPs and specialists being grouped within a same association (the OMA), the medical profession remained divided (more so than in Québec) along political lines. The question of delegating monopoly representation of medical interests to an association was more contentious. Groups of medical doctors voiced more extreme and conservative political positions than the OMA and contested its legitimacy on multiple occasions. In the 1990s, conservative governments in Ontario also criticised the fact that a profession such as medicine would form an association that resembled a workers' union. Some alternative political positions also appeared within the medical profession in Québec across various periods of reforms, but more to support a strong PFHS than pursue a conservative political agenda. In addition, the CMA supported unions and associations as an essential feature of medical politics across Canada. For the CMA, professional associations and unions were an appropriate vehicle to voice the demands of the medical profession so long as governments respected the principles of free negotiations and avoided imposing working conditions by decree. The CMA regarded negotiated agreements a way to promote the medical profession's identification with and attachment to the PFHS.

Medical politics, as expressed within the two Canadian cases, were not produced solely through the medical profession's introspection on their status, roles and working conditions. Cyclical reforms and periods of rationalisation by governments, especially in Québec, inculcated a sense of detachment in the medical profession – of not being sufficiently considered when it came time to think about improving the healthcare system. At the same time, the games played within the mediated space by medical unions and associations likely did not facilitate the development at large scale of joint policy-making between governments and medical doctors. As an institution, medical politics fostered a policy game within the mediated space that tended to be narrow and conflictual. Overall, medical politics appeared as a synthesis of an essentialist view of the profession associated with altruistic values, and a political view of the profession as dedicated to achieving occupational control and protecting its privileges and status.

In England, the creation of a PFHS amplified and formalised the medical profession's perception and conviction that it had to interact with an assertive government eager to take the lead in healthcare policy. Medical specialists were successful in securing their autonomy and gaining significant privileges using traditional channels of influence, that is, their access to political elites. Also, as employees of the PFHS, hospital specialists were more thoroughly integrated into the system. During the first decades after the creation of the PFHS, they were more protected from the intrusion of reformative policies. Governments' reformative efforts were focused on changing the role of GPs, which had only indirect implications on the role of hospital specialists.

As previously noted, medical politics in England were already palpable prior to the creation of the NHS. The medical profession was formally organised and represented through its professional medical union, the BMA. But it was the institutionalisation of the 'double bed' relationship (Klein, 2013) that led to a more structured and strategic approach in the medical profession's dealings with government. The government could no longer ignore the role and influence of medical politics, hence Bevan's choice of an alternative approach to achieving his policy goals. Essentially, medical politics became embedded in the reform process rather than appearing as an exogenous or added factor. This may explain why periods of political turbulence were not as noticeable at the inception of the English PFHS as they were in Québec or Ontario. Medical politics in the English case were also less homogenous, in particular during the first 30 years of the NHS (Webster, 1988; Ham, 2009; Klein, 2013). In contrast, conflicts with governments over the next few decades led the medical profession to resist policy proposals as a unified group, even though the interests of GPs and specialists were not especially aligned. This renewed cohesion of the medical profession was successful in mobilising its professional bodies and union to make its opinion heard inside Parliament. As main providers of healthcare services in England, hospital consultants and GPs consistently defended equality and universality throughout reformative periods as these values went hand in hand with the protection of their professional autonomy (Germain, 2019). Therefore, the medical profession as a whole hardly ever proactively generated significant policy proposals, and for the most part, adopted a reactionary approach to health policy.

Overall, the medical politics we saw in all three cases were as much a legacy from inherited patterns of interaction between governments and the medical profession prior to the inception of the PFHS as an ideological matrix that evolved through experience in the new system. Medical politics, especially in the Canadian cases, became a competing regime of governmentality institutionalised within PFHS. Medical politics influenced the way medical doctors perceived themselves, the way knowledge and expertise became legitimate means to exert power in the PFHS, and the way the medical profession was defined in opposition to policy and managerial initiatives. Within this matrix, regulations, and more broadly, reformative policies, had to align with the political credo of the medical profession.

Confrontation and collaboration within the mediated space of reforms

In the three cases, reforms created a mediated space where government and the medical profession, in a situation of interdependence, became politically active and exerted influence over one another to shape policy changes.

Patterns of interaction observed in the mediated space were influenced by a wide range of contextual factors, including the predominant characteristics of medical politics as an institution, and governments' views on policy-making and the role of the medical profession in PFHS. At times, interactions within the mediated space resonated with broad and transformative socio-political trends such as the promotion of social exchanges and feedback (Campbell, 2011; Blanchet and Fox, 2013; Raine et al, 2014), or co-production in policy design and implementation (Howlett et al, 2017). From a policy-learning standpoint (Howlett, 2012), interactions appeared, over time, to influence and modify the preferences (values, interests and strategic objectives) of our two protagonists. This raised empirical questions around the degree of change in medical politics and government approaches to policy-making. Policy exchanges within the mediated space revealed patterns of interactions that could be defined as predominantly confrontational, collaborative or a mix of both, with different impacts on the evolution of reforms.

Interactions between medical doctors and government within the mediated space varied across our empirical cases. The intensity and dynamics of these interactions appeared to be motivated by a sense of urgency, their respective capacity to influence outcomes and the perceived legitimacy of their interventions (Mitchell et al, 1997). In the period prior to the creation of the NHS, the government crafted a differential strategy that dictated its interactions with GPs and hospital specialists in order to facilitate the adoption of PFHS principles. Although the government felt that it could have acted legitimately on its own, it still wanted to secure the support of medical doctors, and mainly hospital specialists, going so far as offering very substantial financial incentives to assure their cooperation. Members of the political opposition played a role in relaying concerns of the medical profession to government during exchanges on the Bill in the House of Commons (House of Commons, 1946), arguing that Bevan's project would lead to a significant loss of professional autonomy and poor health outcomes. Professional medical bodies, such as the Royal Colleges of Medicine and the BMA, also played a central role in promoting the interests of the medical profession. Financial incentives for hospital specialists, protection of GPs' professional autonomy and limits on State intervention in medical education were granted in exchange for the medical profession's support and collaboration in the PFHS. While this pre-NHS period could have left the medical profession, and particularly GPs, with some residual mistrust in government, it was actually the prelude to a 'golden era' of nearly 30 years of relative harmony.

During the 1960s, GP working conditions in the new PFHS were increasingly perceived as deficient, and this resulted in collective protest through the BMA and threats to withhold services. These tough stances led the government to – slowly and reluctantly –give in to GPs' demands for better compensation. This marked a turning point in the interactions between GPs and the government. The 1970s were characterised by tensions around medical specialists' privileges to treat private patients in public hospitals and their managerial role within the NHS. Through job action and by invoking the premises of the initial 'concordat', medical specialists were able to preserve their key role in the management of the NHS and, with minor concessions, the right to engage in private practice within public hospitals. Patterns of interaction between government and the medical profession became less collaborative, and when issues arose, the medical profession was able to affirm its preferences in the mediated space using hard negotiating tactics such as job action.

During the 1980s and 1990s, a mix of financial constraints leading to the underfunding of the NHS and the emergence of a managerialist ideology culminated in the government adopting a more assertive and confrontational mode of exchange within the mediated space. The government's determination and minimal consultation with the medical profession in the policy formation process significantly changed the dynamics between the protagonists. Despite its relative fragmentation as a political body, the medical profession mounted strong resistance and formed an alliance with the opposition Labour Party. The medical profession realised it had to be active in the mediated space to forge a more tangible, outward-facing identity as a policy-maker. That said, this period ended with the government adopting a more conciliatory approach in order to secure a degree of collaboration from the medical profession and implement the unilaterally developed reforms.

From the end of the 1990s until 2010, a new approach came to the fore, with the Labour government seeking the support of the medical profession to run an ambitious programme of reforms. Although the relationship later deteriorated when the government proved unwilling to concede on working conditions and employment contracts, the early New Labour period was characterised by a return to consensus-based policy-making. The government undertook reforms involving new regulations, market-like mechanisms, financial incentives, clinical governance and performance monitoring (Baggott, 2015). This heterogeneity in policy-making was matched by interactions in the mediated space that oscillated between collaboration and confrontation, which had an impact on the development of medical politics. Professional medical bodies, such as the BMA and the Royal Colleges of Medicine, used different approaches to voice the concerns and preferences of the medical profession during this period, which, to some extent, reduced the influence of the medical profession in the mediated space. The Blair government built on the Thatcher reforms while imposing a modernisation agenda partly motivated and strongly legitimised by scandals around safety and quality of care. The medical profession had no choice but to accept greater government intrusion in its regulation to ensure that professional autonomy would deliver the highest standards of care.

After its election in 2010, the coalition government proposed the introduction of a large-scale reform that aimed to change the role of GPs in the commissioning of healthcare services, giving rise to tense exchanges in the mediated space. Protests from the medical profession as a whole gave rise to opportunistic alliances between the BMA and the Royal Colleges of Medicine that strengthened the profession's resistance to the authoritative imposition of the proposed reforms. Their discontent targeted both the pace and scale of the proposed changes, which had the potential to affect the overall integrity of the PFHS. Finding it difficult to exert authority in the mediated space, the government ultimately handed medical doctors the reins to lead the reform process. The negotiations continued to be difficult and the compromise that was reached masked a political reality where the medical profession had unwittingly returned to an abrasive relationship with government.

Thus, in England we observed a periodic determination by the government to impose healthcare reforms without bringing the medical profession on board. The medical profession, for its part, became more active in the mediated space, explicitly stating its views on reforms and using job action, legal proceedings and public protest to resist the government's reformative ambitions.

We found that the Canadian cases shared some similarities with the English NHS case, but also had unique features. The medical profession adopted an oppositional stance in the period preceding the creation of the PFHS. Medical specialists appeared more strongly opposed to the idea of a PFHS than GPs. Medical doctors in Ontario promoted an alternative type of insurance-based market system and fought to keep control of the fee-for-service compensation system. Contrary to Ontario, where a strong push from the federal government was required to establish the new regime, Québec's government showed more political determination to introduce a PFHS. In both provinces, exchanges within the mediated space between medical doctors and government revolved, from the outset, mainly around working conditions, including extra billing rights (in Ontario), the autonomy of the profession, and the recurring systemic issue of universal access to medical services.

Interactions between our two protagonists in the Canadian cases were shaped by the medical profession's scepticism and mistrust of government. The intensity and dynamics of interactions in these two cases was largely related to contextual factors that had a contingent effect on the relationship between government and the medical profession. Economic constraints or pressure to improve services pushed the government to propose ambitious reforms. In response, medical doctors organised through their unions to fight changes they perceived as undesirable or that threatened their professional autonomy and ability to self-regulate. Interactions in the mediated space followed a pattern whereby the government, mobilising various policy processes, would share reformative ideas and the medical profession would assess these propositions and the risks they presented before developing a proportional strategic response. After periods of intense exchanges that varied depending on the policy issues and context, the government would ultimately accept significant adjustments and propose a compromise that was accepted by the medical profession. This pattern of interactions was less pronounced in Ontario, where the OMA had less legitimacy and a weaker monopoly over representation of the medical profession.

Interaction dynamics appeared more confrontational in the Canadian cases than in the English NHS. Interactions between the medical profession and government were also more frequent and sustained in the Canadian cases. The government appeared more inclined to engage in policy debates with the medical profession and systematically negotiate parts of the reforms that explicitly related to the status and working conditions of medical doctors. Joint policy-making was observed when medical doctors (through their unions, representatives or medical leaders) participated in special bilateral committees established by the government to resolve persistent policy dilemmas. In these situations, the medical profession appeared more engaged in shaping reformative ideas than in the usual bargaining over working conditions. However, the political stance of the medical profession in Canada has typically been more reactive to than generative of health policy proposals. A clear exception to this trend was seen in the policy report *Health Care Transformation in Canada* (CMA, 2010), where the CMA proposed a high-level approach to promoting change in Canadian healthcare systems based on a broad consultation with the CMA membership. In England, the active participation of the BMA and the Royal Colleges of Medicine in policy debates was also primarily reactive rather than generative.

Interaction dynamics between our two protagonists were strikingly context-dependent; however, we were able to identify points of convergence between cases. In all cases, the medical profession took on a more passive role in the resolution of health policy issues, and a more active role when voicing concerns pertaining to working conditions and professional autonomy. The various policy processes and instruments mobilised in all three jurisdictions, including even authoritative instruments such as legal tools, did not appear to impact the manner in which organised medicine became involved and reacted to reformative propositions. In addition, the profession appeared to put more energy into resisting reforms or policy changes than on proposing plausible policy alternatives, with the exception of the bilateral policy-making that took place in formal committee settings. Nonetheless, medical resistance sometimes had a positive influence on the quality of reforms as it raised concerns around inappropriate, misaligned or too-rapid changes. In all three cases, individual medical leaders took part in movements for change, but the collective representative bodies (unions and professional associations) did not seem inclined to act as proactive reformers.

Reforms as becoming: the complexity of change

The outcomes of policy exchanges and interactive dynamics in the mediated space were shaped by a variety of contextual elements: more or less consolidated or unified medical politics, lessons drawn from actors involved in the policy process, and the dynamics established at the inception of the PFHS. Health reforms initiated by government were variably comprehensive and directly impacted to a varying degree on the medical profession. For example, governments in Québec and England were more inclined to launch large-scale health reforms than in Ontario, which, until the late 1990s, favoured incremental policy adjustments over radical interventions. Our study did not aim to assess policy changes or whether reforms improved healthcare system performance, but rather to analyse the influence of the medical profession on the evolution of reformative templates and the nature of adopted reforms.

Because reforms were the result of a constellation of forces, trends and preferences, they usually took the form of a compromise rather than a logical plan that was predictably implemented. Across the cases, we observed variations in the vulnerability of reforms to changes induced by medical politics. Typically, activism led by professional representative bodies tended to focus on elements that directly affected the medical profession's role and status within PFHS. For example, cyclical restructuring of the Québec healthcare system and more modest periods of reorganisation in Ontario received less attention from the medical profession than issues relating to compensation and status. Doctors were not necessarily disinclined to voice their opinion on broader reformative schemes, but tended to limit their interventions to an assessment of proposed policy changes, and often showed distrust in bureaucrats and politicians. In the two Canadian cases, the respective governments seemed able to adopt elements of the reforms that did not appear to directly or predominantly impact the status of medical doctors in healthcare organisations or their working conditions. Medical politics significantly influenced the trajectory of these policies, as revealed by the multiple amendments made to reform proposals in response to medical doctors' concerns. In both Canadian healthcare systems, the creation of the PFHS itself was by far the greatest policy change to directly impact the role of medical doctors and challenge their perspective on medical professionalism. Reforms directly impacting or having the potential to impact medical doctors required a higher level of diplomacy in the negotiated space as they faced the risk of policy dilution and conflict. This was illustrated by the implementation of ad hoc joint policy-making bodies to support such policy changes. These empirical findings were significant across our two Canadian cases and were based on an assessment of medical doctors' reactions to reforms and an analysis of the interactions between government and medical doctors around circumscribed policy changes that related directly to medical doctors.

In England, the medical profession took on the duty to uphold the foundational values of the NHS. Over the years, the profession saw itself as the defender and protector of universality and equity of care. These policy concepts were often used in conjunction with the principle of professional autonomy and independence to halt or radically modify the government's reformative ambitions. Taking a strong defensive stance during the decade-long Conservative rule in the 1980s, the medical profession was successful in taming the government's drive to rationalise healthcare spending and adopt a privately run healthcare system. Similarly, fierce opposition to market-driven reforms proposed by the coalition government in 2010 led to a significant dilution of the final policy package. However, the rhetoric of medical politics should not be naively taken at face value: the medical profession always had a considerable stake in the PFHS, and depicting itself as the ultimate defender of the founding values of the NHS also represented a trump card at the negotiating table.

As seen in Québec and Ontario, the medical profession in England also tended to react more energetically to reforms that impacted medical doctors' compensation and working conditions. However, since reform programmes in England were often more far-reaching than in Canada, they affected the working and pay conditions of the medical profession to a greater extent. Medical professional bodies were therefore virtually always called on to defend the interests of the profession. As pointed out earlier, the status of hospital doctors as public sector employees additionally meant that they had vested interests in healthcare policy initiatives. We also observed that most of the reforms overlapped in time with negotiations over the renewal of contracts, adding a further element of complexity to medical politics. To a certain extent, negotiations over reforms become a tit-for-tat game between our two protagonists. An example of this was the approval, after strenuous negotiations, of a contract agreement in the early 1990s to facilitate implementation of the (toned-down) internal market reforms. The New Labour governments were also keen to keep the medical profession on side by awarding generous financial and working condition benefits in contract renewals. This helped justify the crucial and central role of the BMA in health policy-making in England, as it acted as a representative body both in relation to system-level reforms and in relation to contract negotiations. Perhaps because of this dual role, the professional medical union faced important internal scrutiny and criticism at critical junctures in the development of reform programmes. Unlike the Royal Colleges, which had a unitary mandate, the BMA had the difficult task of carrying out negotiations for both specialists and GPs, and this periodically exposed its shortcomings especially in relation to GPs.

We initially hypothesised that contextual factors would influence the dynamics present within the mediated space and ultimately favour convergence between the reformative agenda of the government and the status, roles and views of medical doctors. Empirically, we observed many instances where changes in context (economic and political cycles, for example) stimulated policy exchanges between government and the medical profession. One of our empirical questions asked how contextual factors would percolate within the mediated space and induce changes in the mindsets of our two protagonists. We also aimed to determine how these factors contributed to modulating policy exchanges in line with reformative templates. While we certainly observed that contextual factors influenced the intensity and dynamics of interactions, these factors did not seem to shape the propensity of medical doctors to engage in proposing reformative ideas.

Generally, in Canada the medical profession was not willing to engage actively with government-led reforms, but this could be because government's did not make a conscious effort to tweak their policy process in favour of more active engagement with the medical profession. In England, however, during the first 30 years, the medical profession willingly took part in the collaborative enterprise that was the NHS, and although it resisted the important structural changes that the Conservative government attempted to impose during the Thatcher era, it reverted to a more cooperative approach with the New Labour government. It was also quick to go back to a more confrontational approach during the coalition government period. More generally, we observed that throughout history, Conservative governments were more ideologically willing to engage in confrontational exchanges with the medical profession than their Labour counterparts that tended to adopt more consensual approaches to healthcare policy-making.

In the Canadian cases especially, governments were progressively captured by the formal labour regimes, leaving three policy pathways accessible. In decreasing order of importance, a first pathway involved exchanges and labour negotiations within the mediated space relating to medical doctors' working conditions and, more marginally, policy innovations. The outcome of these processes was generally a negotiated agreement between the two protagonists or, much less frequently, the imposition by decree of working conditions for medical doctors. This was not dissimilar to the experience of the English NHS, where contractual agreements with hospital specialists and GPs normally resulted from protracted, more or less conflictual, negotiations between government and representatives of the medical profession, the BMA *in primis*. This first pathway privileged incremental changes and a narrow health policy agenda.

A second pathway involved bilateral special committees formed to jointly develop policy options. This appeared promising to push some reforms or policy changes, but was generally difficult to scale up sufficiently to circumscribe the role of the formal labour regime in policy exchanges. Historically, this pathway represented a common approach to policy-making in England, including in healthcare. Thus, the formation of Royal Commissions and ad hoc committees (with the former having a broader remit) was common in the NHS and characterised by strong involvement of the medical profession.

A third pathway, much less visible in our cases, would be through the creation of a reformative partnership between medical doctors and governments. The plausibility of such a political development depends on how broad socio-historical trends around the status of the medical profession and its integration within PFHS and organisations influence policy mindsets and medical politics. This third pathway values joint policy-making and co-production at large scale, and opens up, in principle, to a broader set of innovative policy options. It requires that medical doctors enter the mediated space with strategic projects that intend to shape and regulate the role of medical doctors within PFHS and their connection with other components of the system and broader health policy dilemmas. This last pathway would be a manifestation of the governmentalisation of the State, and is empirically traceable in the implementation of more open but structured policy processes that support the engagement and co-production of medical doctors in health policy.

We only marginally observe this type of policy pathway in the Canadian cases. When governments mobilise, as they did sporadically in Ontario and Québec, key medical leaders in hybrid policy roles, they somewhat align with this third policy pathway. In England, there are limited examples of this policy-making approach, with the *Hospital Plan* of 1962 being perhaps the most significant. The Modernisation Action Teams of the first New Labour government also fall into this category, with the government attempting to mobilise the medical profession. As far as co-optation of key medical leaders, the nomination of Ara Darzi to a key role in government in 2007, and his subsequent review of the NHS, are rather unique in the history of the PFHS.

This detour through the policy pathways that emerge from our empirical findings suggests that the outcomes of reforms are conditioned by multiple changes that arise out of complex policy dynamics and exchanges. Various socio-historical factors enable governments to integrate medical doctors in PFHS to different degrees. Reforms are an opportunity to redefine the relationship between medical doctors and the PFHS, and we see clear differences in the level of integration between the English and Canadian cases. In the end, the outcomes of government interventions and the manifestations of medical politics culminate in the relative capacity to implement large-scale reforms in all jurisdictions and the relative stability of the role played by medical doctors in the healthcare system. The final chapter of the book will look at the theoretical and policy implications of these empirical observations.

6

Discussion and conclusion

Part 1: Research and theoretical contributions
Governance, governmentality and the medical profession
Influence in the mediated space of reforms

Healthcare is central to the functioning of contemporary states, so much so that political scientists have coined the term 'mature healthcare states' (Tuohy, 2012; Ferlie and McGivern, 2013). Our research focuses on the role of medical doctors in reforms within mature healthcare states. Narratives of network governance in the last 30 years highlight governments' inability to achieve policy changes and objectives on their own (Rhodes, 1996; Torfing, 2005). They need the expertise and agency of non-state actors to bring about policy innovations and change. As suggested by Rhodes (1996), *governing without governments* opens up a rich dynamic where state, non-state, traditional and non-traditional policy actors, each with their own projects and preferences, reinvent society. Our research looks at the prospect of joint policy-making in healthcare, focusing on the specific case of the relationship between governments and medical doctors in healthcare reforms.

Tensions and conflict persist in the network narrative of governance, but can, in principle, be transcended by setting up adequate, effective and collaborative modes of governance (Ansell and Gash, 2008). The political and policy *modus operandi* embodied in the network governance narrative is associated with the challenge of achieving consensual politics in a landscape of potentially conflicting preferences, values and interests. Our research empirically probes these tensions and the difficulties of achieving consensual politics while responding to governmental demands for major change. The basic intuition of network governance is that a participatory and open policy process becomes a predominant principle of policy-making in contemporary states as the legitimacy and scope of coercion is reduced. However, this generates the institutional problem of creating convergence among dispersed sets of actors, each of which has its own agency (Meyer, 2010). Our analysis suggests that governments do not easily and consistently invest in renewing policy instruments to overcome challenges associated with distributed agency and the convergence of interests. While the legitimacy of overly relying on coercive approaches in managing healthcare systems remains doubtful, some states like Canada have, over the past few decades, produced a greater number of rules and regulations to support the increasing scope and complexity of government activities (Garant, 2017). This creates additional tensions, but these are not irreconcilable with a participatory policy process. The successive waves of healthcare reform in England reveal similar dynamics, and reflect governments' need to adapt the health system to a diversity of interests and constraints (Hunter, 2016).

Medical doctors are by default part of any significant policy conversation about healthcare policies and health system reforms. The attention paid to the role of medical doctors in healthcare reforms builds on the assumption that they have a special status and position as influential insiders within the health policy ecosystem. Governments contemplating reforms inevitably have to interact and negotiate with medical doctors to bring about change. However, medical doctors often set themselves apart from other professions in modern societies, pointing to their autonomy, recognition and social status. They are privileged interlocutors of governments on medical affairs and health policies but, as we observe, also tend to keep a certain distance and favour selective involvement in reform projects. There are few accounts of how the medical profession interacts with the strategic projects or reforms promulgated by governments (Pollitt and Bouckaert, 2017). In this book, we have carried out an in-depth sectorial analysis of reforms to better understand how the medical profession as an institution intersects and interacts with government in periods of reform. Our initial theoretical frame sees, in reforms, the creation of a mediated space where government and the medical profession exert agency and attempt to influence each other.

Our inquiry offers interesting insights into government's ability to effect changes in sensitive policy areas such as healthcare and to involve medical doctors in this transformative endeavour. Governments are powerful institutions. They have executive powers and valuable resources that can be mobilised in legitimate ways to support policy and legislative capacities (Wu et al, 2015) as well as run ambitious political programmes. Despite reformative discourse promoting a lighter touch (Pollitt and Bouckaert, 2017), most authors would agree that, at least in the Western world, State power has not decreased to the point of becoming an insignificant agent of policy change (Pierson, 2011). However, governments tend to adapt their approach, with more or less determination and success, to support their quest for solutions to collective problems (Pollitt and Bouckaert, 2017). The narratives that proliferate around new modes of governance (Ferlie et al, 2008; Bevir, 2013; Bevir and Waring, 2018) underline the importance of a more diversified and sometimes sophisticated set of policy instruments (Elliott and Salamon, 2002) in leading contemporary policy changes. *Governing with instruments* is part of a call for steering at a distance and influencing non-State actors in their role as *conceptualisers* and *implementers* of policies. Recent work on policy instruments reveals an intimate link between the knowledge and political substrates embodied in these instruments (Lascoumes and Le Galès, 2007). Governments are expected to reinvent policy instruments to deal with conflicting views within the mediated space of reforms. Contextual pressures and the legitimate role of governments in governing PFHS place them in a privileged position to harness the forces of medical politics. To a lesser degree, but in line with the evolution of their professional practices and contingencies, medical doctors are expected to take a more active role in reforms and promote innovative policy instruments with more enthusiasm.

Based on the typology proposed by Schneider and Ingram (1990), we empirically observe the policy instruments that are mobilised within the mediated space by both protagonists to navigate the contested terrain of reforms. Law represents an instrument with high potential for coercion, but governments make limited, or at most, balanced, use of this instrument (see 'Law as an instrument for policy change' of this chapter). In all three empirical cases, we observe within the mediated space a limited ability to achieve joint policy-making between medical doctors and governments. The reformative proposals of governments occasionally reveal a propensity to take pressing challenges seriously and even sometimes mobilise sophisticated policy instruments. The implementation of public commissions or joint committees for policy-making to shape the future of healthcare are examples of learning and capacity instruments that hope to escape the status quo and enrich policy formulation. Symbolic tools or instruments do not appear sufficiently powerful to act on dynamics and exchanges within the mediated space, at least when activated by governments. Appealing to public interests over immediate professional interests (Saks, 2016) is not enough to engage the medical profession in a more collaborative manner in the search for joint solutions. Consensual politics within the mediated space of reforms remains more of an ideal than a reality.

As defined earlier, incentive tools consist of tangible payoffs to induce compliance. Incentives are used as a policy instrument more often in the English case (for instance, the various typologies of commissioning roles for primary care doctors or the clinical leadership drive for change in secondary care) than in the Canadian cases. One may argue that reliance on extrinsic incentives is widespread in both the Canadian and English cases, with money often used to support minimal compliance by medical doctors with healthcare reforms (for instance, when negotiation on doctors' contracts in England overlap with system reform). However, as indicated previously, medical doctors are not a driving force of ambitious reforms in our cases. Manifestations of medical agency are more oriented toward ensuring reforms align with the predominant views of medical professionalism and are coloured by (especially in the Canadian cases) entrenched scepticism about government's role in healthcare. In summary, healthcare reforms appear as a highly contested terrain when they target predominant representations of autonomy and medical professionalism. In such situations, active negotiations tend to weaken reformative proposals and confrontations erode the ability of governments to exploit the full potential of a diversified set of policy instruments.

Looking at the medical profession, we see that medical doctors rely on numerous strategies to promote their viewpoints during reforms. We label the manifestations of these strategies as 'medical politics' to refer to how the profession exerts influence within the mediated space. Analogies between the way the medical profession negotiates reforms and the concept of policy instruments can be made. Medical doctors rely heavily on discursive practices to promote their views of what it means to be a medical doctor and of the risks of letting medical care fall under the control of bureaucrats and rationalisers. These discourses can be seen as symbolic tools. Medical doctors also rely on the strength of their organised representation incarnated in the Canadian cases, and, to a lesser extent, in the English case, by medical unions. The medical union is the instrument of choice, inscribed in law, for the development and implementation of strategies to influence and negotiate reforms within the mediated space. Medical doctors oppose coercive approaches to induce their compliance with reforms. They consider incentives to be better aligned with their attachment to autonomy. We observe in our cases only limited attempts by the profession to strongly promote and rely on capacity and learning instruments in their exchanges with government. However, when these types of instrument are employed, as in joint policy-making around the planning of medical manpower in Québec, both the medical profession and government seem highly supportive of the approach. Efforts to develop and implement a full and sophisticated suite of instruments to support healthcare reforms appear limited, at least with regard to policies that address issues around medical services and the role of medical doctors in PFHS. This situation contributes significantly to the vagaries of reforms.

State and professional identity

Scholars revisiting the Foucauldian concept of governmentality explore how policy instruments can act on identity formation and discourse that become an integral part of any programme of change put forward by modern States. States here are conceived as the origin and bedrock of social relations and consequently of reforms (Lemke, 2007). States delineate what lies within their sphere of influence and what they consider to be private matters (Lemke, 2007). Indeed, modern States are engaged in an ongoing process of change of their own making, relying on a plurality of policy and legal instruments and the indirect use of power that is associated with non-coercive instruments (Waring et al, 2016; Martin and Waring, 2018). The growing interest in pastoral power, and consequently in State strategies that rely on guidance instead of coercion, appears fundamental to expanding joint policy-making. It also implies that governments have an important responsibility for developing a policy process through which joint policy-making with various constituencies, including the medical profession, becomes possible.

In our analysis governments do not appear to rely on differentiated and sophisticated policy instruments to bring the medical profession on board in reforms. A key assumption in the governmentality approach to the State's role in reforms concerns the process of co-determination between the institutionalisation of States and the emergence of historical forms of subjectivation (Lemke, 2007). It is expected that governments, through various techniques (policy instruments, in our case), will create or contribute to new forms of subjectivity that are aligned with their governing objectives, for example by getting medical doctors to actively participate in rationalising the delivery of medical care (Ferlie and McGivern, 2013). In other words, it is expected that modern States will find ways to co-opt and engage the medical profession in reforms, and that the identity of the medical profession within PFHS will evolve and progressively assume responsibility for broader systemic goals. As observed in our cases, reformative discourse often insists on the importance of medical doctors taking a more active role in finding solutions to persistent dysfunctions in PFHS. In this sense, medical doctors have, as non-State actors, a unique position and relationship with government. The creation of PFHS *de facto* establishes them as public sector professionals and, in principle, encourages them to participate in reforms. However, the status of the medical profession, and the political organisations that voice and support its ideological views on the legitimacy and relevance of State interventions in healthcare, restrain medical doctors from being significantly co-opted in the governmentalisation and regulatory projects of States. Medical doctors' resistance to assuming a generative role in healthcare reforms is emblematic of their ability to exert influence in PFHS.

In substantive and normative terms, the grey science of reforms clashes with medical doctors' discourse on professional autonomy and bureaucratic control. The State and the medical profession appear to be a *loose ensemble* (Ferlie and McGivern, 2013), with medical doctors having the capacity to resist governments' reform ambitions or remain passive and limit their engagement in policy-making that goes beyond their immediate concerns. This dynamic varies across our cases, with many situations of explicit resistance by medical doctors in Canada, and an increasing intensity of resistance in England. Looking at the role of medical doctors in reforms raises questions about mechanisms that governments can use to facilitate or promote the compliance of the medical profession with broad reformative objectives. In our cases, political rationalities seem to clash recursively with professional rationalities and the demonstrated ability of the medical profession to engage in resistance (Mumby et al, 2017). Resistance, in most situations, is not focused on the elaboration of counterproposals to solve health system problems. Nor is it productive resistance where medical politics takes the lead in generating policy alternatives to solve collective problems (Courpasson et al, 2012). Medical resistance tends to focus on obtaining additional resources in exchange for a selective uptake of reformative ideas. In our analysis, governments do not significantly impact the mindset of medical doctors with regard to health reforms.

Professional regulation and medical politics

Overall, the rationalisation of medical practice appears as difficult to achieve as the rationalisation of the healthcare system. Tuohy (2018), in her comparative analysis of healthcare systems, notes that: 'Much of the subsequent story of healthcare politics in advanced nations is about the ways in which the medical profession has come to share or cede its position of pre-eminence' (Tuohy, 2018: 42). The question of regulating health professions, including the medical profession, for the public interest is a growing preoccupation across numerous jurisdictions (Saks, 2016; Chamberlain et al, 2018). Governments have developed various strategies to ensure quality and safety of care and to align the expansion of clinical innovation with desirable clinical outcomes (Saltman, 2018). Efforts have been made and have succeeded in most cases to define the necessary credentials to practise medicine, to maintain registers of qualified medical doctors and, with somewhat more difficulty, to remove doctors from practice when needed to protect the public interest (Roche, 2018). Overall, governments in many jurisdictions have been able to intervene to ensure that professional self-regulation is coupled with other mechanisms to make sure that medical doctors are not the sole arbiter of patient needs or societal expectations regarding the quality and safety of care. The expansion of professional regulation opens the principle of occupational closure for discussion, and introduces a more active role for third party scrutiny of the work of medical doctors (Saltman, 2018). Our analysis does not suggest that governments are impotent in regulating the medical profession and ultimately the quality of care and services. Recent analysis of the evolution of the regulation of the medical profession in England (Brown and Flores, 2018), in Canada (Ahmed et al, 2018), and in various other jurisdictions (Dent, 2018) illustrates professional responses to progressively increasing demands for guarantees and safeguards around quality of care. Nevertheless, professional self-regulation is considered less and less sufficient to fulfil expectations for quality, safety and meeting the perceived needs of patients. Professional self-regulation, a core principle of historical and contemporary medical professionalism, is supplemented by systems of clinical governance (Brown and Flores, 2018; Dent, 2018), such as agencies or quality councils (Ahmed et al, 2018), and active involvement of patients in the delivery of care (Pomey et al, 2019; Boutrouille, Régis and Pomey, 2021).

While recognising significant efforts and successes in aligning professional self-regulation and public interest, our analysis reveals that reconciliation between evolving health system imperatives and the preferences of medical doctors – at least those expressed through organised medicine – has been and remains challenging. Regulating the practice of individual medical doctors seems easier than altering the social contract that ties the medical profession to PFHS. Attempts by governments to install the medical profession as a partner to resolve growing systemic tensions between access, quality and cost of care appear more difficult than promoting regulation of the quality of care delivered by individual clinicians. Our analysis of health reforms deals mostly with issues that transcend matters of credentials, registration of qualified practitioners and removal of doctors for malpractice. When these issues appear in our cases, they regard major scandals around malpractice and threats to patient safety that trigger government interest in curtailing the autonomy of the medical profession through greater accountability and additional controls. Our empirical results show that medical politics, based on a specific representation of professional autonomy and a singular reading of the role and added value of governments in healthcare, limit the ability of the medical profession to be an active agent of reform.

Regulating the quality of individual practice appears to be substantively different than changing the nature of the relations between organised medicine and PFHS. Healthcare reforms take a broad look at public interests that call for the adaptation, modernisation and sustainability of PFHS. The role of the medical profession in accommodating these health system challenges appears crucial for the becoming of reforms. In a sense, medical doctors are probably more open to increasing regulation of the quality of individual practice than in striking a new deal that changes the nature of the relationship between the medical profession as a collective and governments within the context of PFHS. In their analysis of the evolution of the regulation of the medical profession in Canada, Ahmed and colleagues (2018) note an evolutionary trend from a neo-Weberian approach to the study of professions that focuses on social and occupational closure as an integral feature of professionalism, to situations where the medical profession as an institution competes with other institutions to define norms and standards that will guide the organisation and delivery of care. As underlined in Chapters 1 and 2 of this book, such an evolutionary trend is coherent with recognition of the growing interdependency between the medical profession and organisations to manage risks and achieve high-quality care. The challenge involves reconciling the development of medical politics with pressures for a new synthesis between professional self-regulation and public interest (see 'Small p and big P: medical politics and healthcare system change' of this chapter).

Consequently, in our study, governments appear relatively weak at influencing the medical profession, and medical doctors seem disinterested in internalising new roles and principles to play a more generative role in reforms. As suggested by Waring and colleagues (2017), the relational dynamics between pastors (the State and its institutions) and their herds (medical doctors), and the roles played by competing discourses or claims (Greenwood et al, 2011), reveal tensions between the governmentality project of the State and the essentialist and autonomist project of medical doctors. In our three cases, medical doctors honour their initial commitment by maintaining their adhesion to the PFHS, but consistently resist the scrutiny of politicians and bureaucratic rationalisers when it goes beyond regulating the quality of individual practice and the competencies of individual practitioners.

While work on the *governmentalisation* of the State (Lemke, 2007) alerts us to the transformative potential of internalisation and subjectivation processes as a way to bring about policy change, in our study these mechanisms do not appear strong enough to contribute to intense and mutual policy learning or to secure medical doctors' compliance with or active involvement in reforms. These mechanisms are not sufficiently robust to enable the development and activation of a wide range of policy instruments conducive to situations of co-production or joint policy-making at a large scale. Our initial theoretical framework also underlines the importance of the law as a consequential contextual variable to shape the exchanges and behaviours of the two protagonists within the mediated space of reforms. The next section explores the role of the law and legal instruments in the reformative process.

Law as an instrument for policy change

The book's empirical findings highlight the prescriptive, and sometimes transformative, role of the law as a core component of the distal and proximal context. Law shapes and organises the relationship between the medical profession and the government. Law provides boundaries for their interaction, and in some instances acts as a driver of health policy change. Governments may rely on legal means to overcome the challenges associated with mobilising medical doctors as active agents of reform. The legal corpus and the way in which law is used across jurisdictions varies, as illustrated in the case studies. Our empirical findings shed light on the manner in which governments, and, to a lesser extent, medical doctors, strategically use legal instruments and institutions to achieve particular objectives. Law is a key contextual factor influencing the negotiation of healthcare reforms. It is also the embodiment of the reform itself, as it formalises the negotiations between government and the medical profession that take place in the mediated space during the reformative process.

In addition, the analysis of legal instruments in England and Canada speaks to the use of coercion and collaboration during the reformative process. It provides a framework with formal boundaries for the interactions between government and the medical profession. The analysis of legislation to enact healthcare policy thus adds a perspective on the formal aspects of the reform process. However, government, the medical profession and the health system are also all governed and regulated by domestic laws that may have an impact on the reformative process and the formalisation and implementation of healthcare reforms. Legal analysis thus complements the policy and organisational perspective to make sense of the constraints and tools at the disposal of the two protagonists.

In both the Canadian and English systems, interests and values shape the agreement reached between the medical profession and the government in establishing a system and framing its organisation. In England and in Canada, the medical profession accepts the State's egalitarian approach to free and universal access to care in exchange for the preservation of professional autonomy. These values provide the foundations of a 'bargain' or 'concordat' between the medical profession and the government that is formalised in law in Canada and remains tacit in England. Our empirical findings show that this initial agreement, and its particular characteristics in each jurisdiction, plays a pivotal role in structuring the relationship between the medical profession and government in subsequent reformative periods.

The prescriptive dimension of the law has a substantial impact on the manner in which the medical profession is able to assert its position in the mediated space. In England, because of the nature of legal sources and the history of uncodified constitutional rules, law plays a different but equally crucial role in healthcare reforms. Indeed, the non-codified nature of the constitutional legal corpus and the rules around parliamentary democracy give governments strategic leverage. The government's bargaining power in health policy stems from the non-formalised agreement it has with the profession. For instance, rules and customs around who may interact in legislative institutions structure the interactions between the medical profession and government. MPs debate Bills in the House of Lords or House of Commons without the presence of stakeholder groups (Besly et al, 2018). The medical profession, therefore, must find alternative channels, whether professional medical associations such as the Royal Colleges of Medicine or their union (the BMA), to lobby MPs to relay their views on reform proposals (Klein, 2013). Although the medical profession may be invited to comment on White Papers before the legislative process is initiated, it may only be indirectly involved in the formal rule-making process.

In essence, the tacit agreement established in the original NHS Act 1946 defines an implicit role for the medical profession due to the nature of labour and industrial relations in England, and a more explicit role featured in some of the major NHS acts analysed in this book. In contrast with Canada, medical professionals in England are not party to any explicit formal agreement with the government that helps them assert their position during negotiations around the organisation or financing of the health system. Our findings suggest that the British government thus has greater discretion in setting the terms and conditions of medical doctors' role in the health system. The specific rules governing interactions in legislative institutions also give government the choice of whether or not to consider the medical profession's position.

In the Canadian cases, the formal role and recognition given to medical unions negotiating on behalf of the medical profession gives them substantial leverage in healthcare reforms. Medical unions are guaranteed a seat at the negotiating table for policy shifts or reforms that may impact the medical profession. Government and medical unions are bound by laws – by the Québec Charter, for instance (the Canadian Charter only applies to government) – that establish the parameters of negotiations and may curtail certain pressure tactics or policy options.

Governments (particularly majority governments) are in a strategic position when mobilising legislative power to put forward reformative bills that may be fully or partially adopted by Parliament. Such instruments are used to create incentives or as tactics for coercion. In instances where agreement cannot be reached, governments may try to coerce medical doctors into specific actions by adopting a law; we see special laws adopted in response to specific actions by the medical profession, for instance to end a strike. Governments also use the legislative process strategically to gain traction, with omnibus Bills (covering a number of diverse or unrelated topics, subject to a single vote by the legislature) or by limiting the consultation period on reformative bills (as in the Barrette reform in Québec).

Medical doctors in Canada can also rely on legal tools to gain traction in negotiations or launch legal proceedings to contest the validity of laws (for example, the Canada Health Act); they often abandon the proceedings when a settlement with government is reached. In Canada, the medical profession's preservation of autonomy and reluctance to comply with reformative ambitions may be attributable to the fact that it has more legal instruments at its disposal (although fewer than government) to negotiate and partially neutralise the government's coercive power.

The courts have at times forced the hand of governments and medical doctors, requiring them to change their practices to comply with fundamental rights (for instance, in the *Chaoulli* and *Fédération des médecins spécialistes du Québec vs Conseil pour la protection des malades* cases in Québec).

Across reformative periods, our empirical findings reveal that governments often threaten but rarely follow through with the imposition of legislation to force reforms, potentially because they know this would make it more difficult to secure medical doctors' support ex post. Governments therefore tend to negotiate and renegotiate reforms instead of imposing them. The risk of long and costly legal battles is another deterrent to government use of legal instruments.

The procedural and substantial role of law in England was also relevant to our analysis in various aspects. The boundaries imposed by England's law and rule-making process structure relationships in a way that has a significant impact on the reformative process. In the Canadian context, despite the availability of multiple legal instruments, the medical profession remains more reluctant to comply with reformative ambitions and has preserved its autonomy in the system. This may be because medical doctors also have more legal instruments at their disposal (although fewer than government) to negotiate and partially neutralise government's coercive power. The risk of long judicial battles, with their ensuing costs to both sides, and especially in terms of the subsequent success of reforms, may exert a chilling effect on government.

While the legal context at times percolates into the mediated space and shapes the nature of exchanges between medical doctors and government, we observe an overall reluctance on the part of governments and medical doctors to rely on legal instruments. Factors such as the nature of the policy shift and a government's leadership style (collaborative or authoritative) influence the use of legal instruments. Coercion is not the preferred option. A government relying heavily on legal tools (laws, regulation and enforcement mechanisms) to influence healthcare may develop a form of instrumental legal leadership that impacts negatively on medical doctors' willingness to comply with the objectives of a reform (Tyler, 2011). Such leadership also diverges from the tendency in recent years to diversify the set of policy instruments that embody less coercive approaches.

In the two previous sections, we have revisited our empirical findings using theoretical frameworks from scholarly works on new modes of governance, governmentality and law. We conclude that medical doctors participate in reforms by complying with negotiated agreements in line with their own strategic predispositions. Compliance is achieved under constraints imposed by a specific representation of autonomy, professionalism and legal options. Signs of change in the internalisation of a new representation of medical professionalism and subjectivities towards new roles in reforms are only vaguely apparent in the manifestations of medical politics in our cases. This is our understanding of the medical profession's adoption of a socially conservative agenda. Medical doctors' professional project has adopted a defensive position that seems effective at promoting their views, interests and values in reforms. The reforms are, in many instances, the product of a policy compromise or a series of accommodations that constrain the States' ability to solve crucial policy dilemmas. The following section deals with potential changes in medical politics, exploring the prospect of a new relationship between the medical profession and healthcare organisations that has emerged in PFHS. While change appears difficult between medical doctors and the State, change does, in fact, occur at organisational level.

Small p and big P: medical politics and healthcare system change

The medical profession is considered an ideal-type professional archetype (Freidson, 1974). As we observe empirically, medical doctors rely on a specific interpretation of professionalism and institutional mechanisms to assert their views and interests. While this is akin to an essentialist conception of the profession that fully aligns with altruistic values (Parsons, 1954), medical politics also seems at times to resist interference from government that promotes broader societal values such as equitable access to care. This is more evident in the Canadian cases than in England. As presented in our theoretical chapter (Chapter 2), studies on the interface between organisations and professions (Leicht and Fennell, 1997), including healthcare organisations (Kitchener et al, 2005), suggest that the medical profession, like other professions, proceeds with incremental changes when organisational imperatives infiltrate its professional ethos and *modus operandi* (Noordegraaft, 2011). Medical doctors do not oppose organisational demands, but seek to simultaneously achieve a professional and organisational project. Increased complicity and accommodation has been observed and predicted in studies on organisational professionalism and in concepts such as professional communities where collaboration is the mechanism through which professional values and interests are reconciled with organisational goals (Adler et al, 2008). Our study does not focus on this level of analysis, but we logically expect that changes at organisational level will have repercussions on the project promoted by medical politics at a more macro level. However, we do not empirically observe significant permeability with changes cutting across organisation and policy levels.

Recent work on organisational fields (Zietsma et al, 2017) in neo-institutional analysis suggests that they are key elements in the formation of modern political and organisational life. While their review distinguishes between broader societal and organisational fields, Zietsma et al (2017) suggest that fields are organised around a more or less elaborated institutional infrastructure and various levels of agreed prioritisation among actors. A field's institutional infrastructure refers to 'the mechanisms of social coordination by which embedded actors interact with one another in predictable ways' (Zietsma et al, 2017: 392). Agreed prioritisation is defined as actors in situations of competing institutional logics that tend to converge towards predominant logics. The example of professional exchanges in a field is used to illustrate situations where, as in the case of medicine, the profession consistently espouses a relatively homogeneous logic – for example, their views on professional autonomy and control – even if they have to exchange with a variety of entities including governments and other health professions. Persistence in agreed prioritisation is certainly a feature of the views promulgated within the mediated space of reforms. It is part of the institutional work performed by medical doctors to accommodate changes while staying aligned with deeply engrained values.

Our analysis does not focus on delineating the boundaries or nature of the professional field of medicine, but rather on the conditions that make a profession engage with a specific type of change that we label reforms. Insights provided by neo-institutional work in organisational fields suggest that the medical profession will progressively and actively strike a new balance between its preferences and the preferences dictated by organisational and societal needs and demands. In addition, the proliferation of works on the evolution of professional mindsets and behaviours within organisations, and on the role of professions as agents of institutional change (Muzio et al, 2013), lead us to expect exchanges and politics in the mediated space to exhibit more voluntarism towards change on the part of the medical profession. The intense exchanges around reforms would induce learning where competing institutions and logics attempt to redefine healthcare and the role of medical doctors within the institution of PFHS. Our empirical findings suggest that while accommodations may occur on a day-to-day basis in healthcare organisations, this has not significantly infiltrated medical politics that play out at systemic level. The changes that occur at the organisational level, broadly defining this field as encompassing educational institutions in shaping the profession as an institution, do not significantly influence the manner in which organised medicine and government interact and shape health policies. In our cases, the medical profession does not, in most situations, embrace the role of active agent of institutional change in the context of healthcare reforms.

A possible explanation for this lies in the way exchanges between the medical profession and governments are formally structured in the context of PFHS. We see differences between the two countries. In England, the initial deal embodies an implicit agreement whereby medical doctors accept becoming an integrated component of the new system. We thus see in England some greater involvement of medical doctors in enacting reforms In Canada, negotiations around the creation of the PFHS cement the insider–outsider status of the medical profession. Medical doctors see themselves as such, and governments accept this state of affairs. Medical doctors participate in PFHS without having much formal responsibility for the functioning and maintenance of the system beyond their immediate clinical duties. This is not to say that, on an individual basis, medical doctors do not contribute to PFHS, but the initial agreement somewhat precludes them from being an agent of institutional adaptation and change.

The medical profession occupies a different position in each country and in each PFHS. However, variations in the legal instruments available in a jurisdiction do not significantly impact the profession's propensity to engage actively with change. Medical politics in England and Canada share features such as the definition of professional autonomy and scepticism of government policy changes. In all three cases examined in this book, the medical profession is organised around a relatively fragmented political body. Frequently, the interests of medical specialists and GPs are misaligned or antagonistic. Fragmented medical politics may impede institutional work towards a more contemporary version of medical professionalism. Also, the socially conservative agenda of the medical profession, encompassing a high degree of scepticism for government intervention, has limited the medical profession's ability to actively engage in reforms. In mature healthcare states, the medical profession has simultaneously resisted reformative projects and found it difficult to assemble the political conditions to fully and genuinely participate in the State's regulatory enterprise. Fragmented medical politics are associated with a less generative role in healthcare reforms. Our analysis of medical politics as an institution and agent of change finds that joint policy-making between government and medical doctors has played little role in reforms.

In summary, based on our theoretical framework and empirical analysis, we are surprised to observe how resilient and stable the initial agreement between the medical profession and government at the inception of the PFHS remains across time and somewhat predetermines the nature of exchanges within the mediated space of reforms. As underlined by neo-institutionalists, health policy in the making is a game between competing institutions and logics, in this case the profession and government. At the outset of this research, we expected to see more blurring of boundaries between systems of meanings and logics that drive positioning, exchanges and tactics within the mediated space of reforms. In fact, the greatest change we observe in our analytical journey is the initial one, namely, the creation of PFHS. The creation of PFHS represents a unique achievement where governments are able to address imminent challenges and societal needs, but also forge compromises among competing forces to make possible the creation of a new institution. From the onset of PFHS, a long process of maturation and consolidation, unfolding with various intensity in our two jurisdictions, takes place and gives rise to the institution of medical politics as a bedrock of contemporary health systems. Learning occurs, but does not really facilitate a new synthesis among competing institutions and logics. Learning takes place by adapting the role of government as regulator and by reinforcing the role of the medical profession as inside influencer.

Part 2: Policy implications

Medical doctors are inside influencers in PFHS. By accepting to join PFHS, they become unavoidable actors. Moreover, in their day-to-day work, they influence the utilisation of resources within PFHS. In a survey of medical doctors in the US, Gruen et al find that many in the profession support a role that goes beyond usual clinical duties:

> Our findings suggest that many medical doctors believe they have professional responsibilities to healthcare-related issues outside their direct clinical practice, and that these are considered to be responsibilities of individual physicians, expressed through community participation and individual political involvement, as well as of their professional associations. These findings are consistent with a view of professionalism in which medical doctors are responsible in their areas of expertise to contribute to helping the society that grants them professional status. If medical doctors subscribe to this view, then they likely perceive a point where their responsibilities as experts end, and their civic responsibilities are no greater than those of other members of societies. (Gruen et al, 2006: 2473)

Medical doctors appear open to roles that extend beyond traditional views of medical professionalism. Engagement with broader health system issues is supported, but in more immediate or community spaces. In their analysis of primary healthcare reforms in Canada, Strumpf and colleagues (2012) conclude that GPs are more inclined to consider alternate models of care and reforms that are incremental and characterised by voluntary participation. In Canada, medical doctors engage in various ways and at various scales in clinical networks and improvement initiatives (see, for example, the case of Strategic Clinical Networks in Alberta in Yiu et al, 2019). The engagement of medical doctors in activities and roles that go beyond normal clinical duties is possible when these are directly related to their communities or practice settings. This reveals the importance of framing reforms in a way that has meaning to the practice experience of medical doctors and other professionals. Multiple studies have documented aspects of medical doctors' engagement within their clinical, organisational and community contexts (Kaissi, 2014; Dickinson et al, 2016).

The experience of reforms in England also suggests that primary care doctors are more willing to engage with different models of care. From the creation of the purchasing role with GP fundholding in the 1990s, to the emergence of commissioning organisations (PCTs in the 2000s and especially CCGs in 2012) and, more recently, the introduction of networks (PCNs) of GP practices, GPs (at least a sizeable proportion of them) have repeatedly demonstrated their readiness to accept roles and responsibilities beyond their traditional clinical duties. This has also included the creation of multi-specialist practices and community services. Conversely, specialist doctors have generally been far less willing to go beyond the boundaries of acute care settings or even their individual specialties, with some exceptions such as Cancer Care Networks.

Our study deals less with the engagement of medical doctors at an individual or group level (within organisations or practice settings) than with their engagement as a constituency that can play a role in shaping healthcare system policies. This broader level of engagement is in essence more macroscopic and more political. It implies the active participation of political bodies that represent or are associated with the medical profession in the formulation of policies to cure healthcare system dysfunctions and vulnerabilities. It also implies an ability in the medical profession to create a degree of political unity within its ranks to promote desirable policy changes. As inside influencers, medical doctors cannot be ignored in forging healthcare reforms. Governments and the medical profession face the challenge of creating collaboration at scale to shape the destiny of PFHS. Our empirical findings show variations in the integration of the medical profession within PFHS; England and Canada represent an interesting contrast in this respect, but in both national contexts, the medical profession assumes a relatively passive role in advocating for reforms. Policy ideas to transform PFHS do not take root in a significant way within the medical profession. Medical doctors, at least through the voice of organised medicine, are more reactive and protective than active proponents of change.

This situation raises the question of what can be done to bring medical doctors on board in reforms and make them allies in a transformative journey at the policy level. Our empirical findings provide some insights. To start with, the institutional substrate that enables and constrains relations between medical doctors and governments matters. We observe through time in both Canadian cases a growing role for labour regimes in the mediated space of reforms. Labour regimes become a privileged setting in which the roles of the medical profession in the improvement of PFHS are considered and debated. This situation has three main implications. First, it tends to compress the definition of policy issues into elements that are negotiable within labour regimes. The question of medical compensation almost inevitably becomes a centre of gravity when it comes to translating policy objectives into acceptable policies for the medical profession. This is, as we have seen, more salient in the Canadian cases. However, despite different employment arrangements in England, we observe similar struggles to achieve joint policy-making when the formulation of health policies overlaps with negotiations over contractual arrangements. Discussions over the direction of the PFHS and priority setting become entangled with arguments over compensation packages and working conditions. Often, the introduction of significant reforms is sweetened by favourable financial treatment and preservation of autonomy. These transactional aspects appear as a necessary condition for transformational intentions. It clearly suggests the importance of supplementing policy exchanges between governments and medical doctors with others policy opportunities and arenas. In both countries, instances of joint policy-making are observed empirically and occur alongside the rigid processes associated with predominant labour regimes. Experiences of more collaborative policy-making through various convening strategies initiated by both protagonists appear productive and suitable. Clearly there is a need for government to be better equipped to create such opportunities and negotiate a broader policy space in which medical doctors can engage in reforms. But it also depends on the willingness of medical doctors to engage beyond the boundaries of narrow 'iron cage' professional interests.

Second, while there is a growing and legitimate interest in the engagement of medical doctors within their practice and community settings, there is also a need to intervene at the level of the predispositions of medical doctors when they enter the profession and, more importantly, as they practise medicine. Medical doctors in the Canadian cases and in England appear relatively silent about the limitations imposed by medical politics, as revealed by the discourse and practices of their unions or professional associations. Beyond what we have already identified as policy opportunities, governments and professional bodies such as colleges and institutions of higher education must engage much more actively in socialising medical doctors to embed their practice within the PFHS. PFHS offer the medical profession many opportunities in terms of resources for their practice, and medical doctors in their daily practice provide a whole range of services and expertise to the healthcare system and their patients. It is important to involve them in broader healthcare system issues and frame and mobilise medical politics as a constructive force in system change. Policy forums where various medical bodies and governments exchange views and ideas can be productive. Determination is needed on both sides to build the capacity to structure such exchanges. Again, professional bodies and institutions of higher learning can play a crucial role. Potential positive outcomes include not just the socialisation of the medical profession to broader system issues, but also greater government and policy-maker understanding of the positions and responsibilities of medical doctors. It is no accident that one of the most enduring policy drives in the English NHS – the emergence of clinical leadership 'from the dark side to centre stage' (Ham et al, 2011) – is the result of a policy mandate framed by a prominent clinician, Ara Darzi (Secretary of State for Health, 2008). Finding ways to increase the odds of policy innovations is crucial to achieve reforms.

Third, governments and the medical profession must recognise the limitations imposed by bilateral policy exchanges within the mediated space of reforms. Policy experiments such as public commissions have been used to generate policy ideas in Québec at key points in the evolution of the PFHS. There is a challenge in moving from bilateral to multilateral exchanges where other health professions, health managers and civil society actors get involved in a common mediated space and influence each other. This seems important to influence predispositions and work on a mutual understanding of problems and solutions. Reforms are too often debated in a very fragmented way while policy innovations are needed that support the *systemness* property of PFHS (Lewis, 2015). Our empirical findings suggest that governments and the medical profession in Canada engage in policy debates around reforms in a very confined space that increases the risk of conservatism. Recent agreement between the Québec government and the specialist medical union (FMSQ) to create an institute on the appropriateness of medical care (Institut de la pertinence des actes médicaux, IPAM; see https://ipam.ca) coupled with financial incentives will be interesting to follow. The deeper question that needs to be asked is about the possibility of engaging the medical profession in transformative policy work within the confined space of medical politics and organised medicine.

The experience in Canada is not dissimilar to what we see in England. Traditional fora such as Royal Commissions can garner a broader policy consensus, but can also be limited in their remit and in how they influence the subsequent policy-making process. Another example could be the Modernisation Action Teams of the New Labour period, which were put together to facilitate wider participation in policy formulation. Another approach might be to provide broad policy frameworks and let the main actors in the system fill in and adjust the contours, as is seen with the establishment of PCNs in the 2019 *NHS Plan*. The policy mandate does little more than introduce these new, loose organisational forms and provide financial incentives for GP practices to join. Such bottom-up, collaborative organisational forms require time and resources, and expectations around the pace of change must be adjusted accordingly.

Ultimately, in our study, it appears clear that the roles of medical doctors cannot be understood without paying attention to the roles played by government in promulgating and negotiating reforms. Governments are payers and have significant stakes in ensuring a sustainable, effective and well-functioning healthcare system. They tend to be hyperactive in promoting reforms, yet very modest in their determination to reinvent policy exchanges with the medical profession. The medical profession also appears very conservative about engaging significantly and differently in the policy change journey. In the end, both governments and medical doctors participate in their own way in so-called healthcare reforms. They engage in conflicts and harsh negotiations at times, but in the end are neither allies nor enemies in reforms. They both continue along their way and show limited ability to change the policy game.

Our study reveals the importance of a granular analysis of the evolution of the roles of medical doctors in contemporary healthcare policies. It involves two mature healthcare states. Similar analysis needs to be performed on other countries characterised as mature healthcare states that have more pluralist healthcare systems, such as France, the Netherlands and Germany. In addition, our study does not consider the evolution of public professions in healthcare, such as the nursing profession. The role of the nursing profession in healthcare policies and reforms needs to be better understood on its own, and as it interacts with the medical profession in policy-making. Finally, more attention needs to be paid to alternate policy approaches based on the principle of joint policy-making, and the implications of these approaches for the trajectory of healthcare reforms.

Epilogue

As an epilogue, we completed this analysis just before the COVID-19 pandemic. We have since been able to observe the commitment and dedication of front-line clinicians, medical doctors and others healthcare professionals and workers in dealing with extraordinary and immense pressure to deliver care, often at considerable risk to their own health. In a sense, the commitment of medical doctors confirms one of the key findings of our study: the discrepancy between medical politics and the day-to-day accommodation between the medical profession and the healthcare system. It is self-evident that healthcare systems would greatly benefit if the dedication and willingness seen in clinical matters could percolate to policy level decision-making. This is the main reason we stress that joint policy-making is not just a responsibility of medical doctors, but also of governments that need to find a way to adequately mobilise medical doctors at a collective or policy level.

Beyond this, COVID-19 has become part of the distal context that could trigger policy shifts and radical healthcare reforms. This major public health crisis has created a significant burden on government finances, led to an important reorganisation of resources in healthcare systems – including the delay of essential care such as cancer treatments – and generated an extra burden on some healthcare professionals now facing increased fatigue and burnout (Denning et al, 2021; Gemine et al, 2021). It has also revealed how painfully inadequate healthcare systems have become in dealing with public health issues. In this sense, the pandemic has exacerbated vulnerabilities that were already present in the Canadian and English health systems, notably with respect to the elderly population living in long-term care facilities (Estabrooks et al, 2020; Hinsliff-Smith et al, 2020) and more vulnerable segments of the population such as minority ethnic communities, women and homeless people (National Housing Federation, 2020; Women and Equality Committee, 2020; Germain and Yong, 2021a; Henry et al, 2021). More broadly, it is clear that the effects of the pandemic have been most significant in communities that were already at a disadvantage due to structural inequalities (Health Foundation, 2020; Germain and Yong, 2021b; forthcoming). This COVID-19 context will undoubtedly leave a footprint on PFHS that we can currently barely fathom.

How much the pandemic experience will be transformative and what impact it will have on the medical profession and on the relationship between medical doctors and government is an evolving question. Governments and medical doctors will have to deal with major issues in the aftermath of the pandemic such as restoring essential care. In England, for instance, the significant backlog of procedures and treatments has reached unprecedented levels (more than 5 million people on waiting lists, as of April 2021). While governments face serious shortfalls in public finances, the urgency of recuperating capacities and pressure to offer decent access to essential healthcare services places the medical profession in an advantageous position. Medical doctors will play a key role in resuming service and restoring full capacity in health systems. Other health workers who played a crucial role during the pandemic are now advocating for recognition in the form of better compensation (Denis et al, 2021). The aftermath may bring about conditions for a new and more collaborative deal across professions and between the professions and government in Canada. However, in England the government has already outlined its position, granting a 3 per cent pay increase to NHS staff after initially proposing a meagre 1 per cent (Walker et al, 2021). Within the medical profession, the lack of national guidance to deal with this unprecedented crisis may leave the profession less receptive to government ambitions. All these elements are likely to have an impact on the expression of medical politics and its contribution to healthcare reforms.

The COVID-19 pandemic also shed light on the unexpected agility of the Canadian and English healthcare systems to organise successful vaccination campaigns. Both health systems have also shown a capacity to redeploy their workforce and make better use of telemedicine and remote consultations (Bhatia et al, 2021). The pandemic also brought to the fore the importance of public health. For many years, clinical care has been the dominant theme of reforms and the main recipient of financial investments, arguably due in part to the key role of medical doctors in the negotiating space. For example, not long ago in Québec, Health Minister Gaétan Barrette stated that he did not understand what public health had to do with the healthcare system and significantly reduced public health spending (Fiset-Laniel et al, 2020). England has seen years of disinvestment in the infrastructure and resources needed for effective public health provision. The experience of the COVID-19 pandemic makes it impossible to pretend that public health is not worthy of more attention in healthcare systems, although the abolition of Public Health England in the middle of the pandemic does not help understand what to expect in future. Furthermore, there is an inherent tension between putting money towards healthcare and investing in improving the health of the population. These questions and expectations will be part of the post-pandemic context, will nurture debate over where to put resources in and around PFHS, and may impact the manifestation of medical politics in health system changes.

Ultimately, the key challenge for governments and healthcare systems will be to organise the post-pandemic period. Ideally, this rebuilding phase will allow for a thoughtful process of defining the lessons learned in order to build on them. Key avenues of reform will most likely consist of restructuring the long-term care sector, redefining on a medium- and long-term horizon the contribution of public health and the role of primary care in a modern PFHS, including greater recognition of healthcare professionals working in this area. Governments will face the challenge of balancing the role and contribution of clinical services versus public health. Governments will also have to decide which 'agility outputs' deserve to be permanently integrated into healthcare systems, knowing that finances will be on a tight leash. Governments will probably build on the new openness to telemedicine and remote care to push implementation of digitalised medicine. Innovation may become a new credo in PFHS. The institution of professions, and more specifically the institution of medical politics, will be a central piece in the implementation of a post-pandemic innovative agenda within PFHS.

Interestingly, some of the changes triggered in the post-pandemic phase might also become necessities more than options due to intervention by the courts. As the dust settles, there will be a period when governments must answer in the judiciary arena for some of the choices they made during the crisis. This explanatory process has already started (see, for instance, *Clinique juridique itinérante c. Procureur général du Québec*, 2021, QCCS 182), but will likely increase when the urgency abates. In England, calls for a public inquiry into the government's response to the pandemic have grown louder by the day. At the time of writing, NHS organisations have been told to retain all relevant documents ahead of an imminent inquiry. The legal community will push to require accountability, reparations or changes from actors who made decisions during the crisis. The courts may be deferential to government actions considering the complexity of the pandemic, the difficult resource allocation choices that had to be made and the evolving scientific evidence. Nevertheless, courts will require explanations and, in some circumstances, transformations that will force governments and healthcare actors such as medical doctors to adapt to rectify courses of action they took during the pandemic. The situation in long-term care facilities is an area the courts will not let pass considering the major impact it had on people's life, liberty and safety. A return to the old ways in this area seems improbable.

While at first sight our empirical findings suggest a rather pessimistic assessment of the role of medical doctors as a force of change in PFHS, emerging trends in medical politics may provide the basis for a more positive rendering. A recent report by the CMA advocates for an ambitious programme of changes to achieve integration of care, equity and better population health within the context of PFHS and in the aftermath of the pandemic (CMA, 2021). It calls for bold reforms to rapidly take advantage of the windows of opportunity opened by the experience of the pandemic. The report is about medical politics with a very progressive and transformative twist, inviting the active participation of medical doctors in improving and transforming PFHS without undermining the system's legitimacy. This report clearly positions medical doctors as concerned inside influencers who aspire to changes that go far beyond the conservative social agenda associated with medical politics observed in our empirical research. This report is a policy statement at national level. A similar activation of medical politics in the aftermath of the pandemic must also occur at sub-national levels in Canada in order to be truly transformative.

In England, the absence of clear national guidance during the pandemic on how to ration and allocate resources to deal with the surge in patients in primary and secondary care settings left the medical profession no choice but to assume a more active policy role. During the first months of the pandemic, the BMA and Royal Colleges of Medicine issued guidance for front-line clinical staff on how to deal ethically with the allocation of resources for patient care, personal protective equipment and human resources (BMA, 2020; RCP, 2020). However, instead of seizing the opportunity to make bold propositions, these professional medical organisations fell back on existing frameworks to structure their guidelines. This may be explained by the fact that the NHS was on the brink of being overwhelmed and medical professionals took on the role of drafting guidance on top of heavier clinical duties. In this respect, the public health crisis did not mark a radical change in the medical profession's role in healthcare policy-making (Germain, 2021). Other issues relating to barriers to accessing healthcare services were exacerbated during the pandemic and have heightened the need for reform initiatives that have been brewing for some time (Germain and Yong, 2020). These stem in part from insufficient integration within the healthcare sector and between health and social care, cumbersome procurement rules, and skill shortages in the healthcare workforce. Building on existing proposals from NHS England aiming to create a stronger and more effective integrated care system, in February 2021 the government announced a White Paper focusing on integration and innovation in health and social care (Department of Health and Social Care, 2021). The policy proposal aims to facilitate collaboration and integration across providers by reversing changes introduced with the Health and Social Care Act 2012. This includes removing rules on competition and procurement to increase flexibility and facilitate place-based partnerships. Unusually for a Conservative-led reform, it intends to increase central power over the NHS by strengthening ministerial control over the day-to-day running of the healthcare system, empowering the Secretary of State to direct NHS England in relation to formal functions. Disappointingly, considering the disproportionate impact of the pandemic on the sector, it lacks a detailed plan for social care reform, mentioning only stronger central oversight and more limited funding for providers. The House of Commons Health and Social Care Committee has already requested greater clarity in this area. The policy proposal is also silent on strategies to solve chronic staff shortages. In terms of structural arrangements, CCGs will be dismantled with their responsibilities transferred to Integrated Care Systems (ICS). As loose reproductions of the US Accountable Care Organization (ACO) model, these umbrella organisations are already part of the NHS, but will now formally become statutory bodies and will pursue integration within the NHS through strategic planning and resource allocation decisions, including commissioning. Other ICS will focus on integration with local stakeholders via broad partnership roles and delegated budgets. The reform would not spell a complete end to commissioning, but would certainly bring the NHS back to a pre-1991 arrangement.

Again, following the trend of previous reform periods, the role of the medical profession in this latest proposal has been rather subdued. The BMA's first reaction was to question the timing of the proposal and vindicate a central role for clinicians in any plan for NHS reform (BMA, 2021). The abolition of post-2012 structures and competition rules is seen positively, but there is great concern about the Secretary of State's 'power grab' over the health service. In fairness, the medical profession has, for some time, strongly supported the principle of integrated care, and hence a move in this direction appears to align with the views and interests of the profession. Nevertheless, there is also concern that the engagement and involvement of clinicians will not be at the heart of the future system, leading to a decrease in clinical leadership currently represented by GP-led CCGs. New commissioning functions will have to be paired with adequate levels of scrutiny. Importantly, medical doctors have emphasised that greater attention should be paid to increasing the safety of NHS staff and upgrading skills in the workforce. This is line with recommendations made by the House of Commons Health and Social Care Committee. Additionally, the BMA has been quick to point out in no uncertain terms that the independent contract status of GPs is not up for discussion.

Appendix: Key constructs and related concepts

Constructs and concepts	Definition	Empirical assessment
Accountability	Evolving expectations of clarity, transparency and responsibility from medical doctors or governments towards goals or tasks achievements. Rewards or sanctions may result from met or unmet expectations.	Identify statements about targets, transparency, duties and responsibilities, performance management and the implication of these statements for the medical profession.
Agency	Generic and generative that focuses on the actions at a collective level from governments and medical doctors in the context of reforms. Such actions aim at demonstrating reflections in regard to their positions and development of appropriate and related strategies.	Identify specific actions and strategies taken by governments and medical doctors within each phase of reforms. Manifestation of agency can be detected from various sources. For instance, a Position Paper by a medical association or an explicit act of opposition from the medical profession to a proposed piece of legislation, or even the use of new policy instruments by the government to influence medical doctors.
Agreements	The act or fact of achieving consensus through formal or informal arrangements and tools (eg, contracts, settlements, joint statements, partnerships, etc).	Identify statements that reflect explicit adhesion or support to the content of reform or some parts of a reform. Agreement also relates to support by both parties on process elements to settle divergence around reforms or explore policy options (for example, creation of an advisory committee composed of representatives of the government and the medical profession).
Alliance	Ad hoc or established coalition between healthcare actors with common values, interests or purpose.	Identify set of individuals, groups or organisations sharing a similar position in regard to the content and the process of a reform.

Constructs and concepts	Definition	Empirical assessment
Autonomy	The manner in which the agency of the profession is related to the expression of some values. Agency builds on autonomy and can be deployed to defend and protect autonomy. Self-regulation, entrepreneurship and collegiality are markers of autonomy for the medical profession.	Identify references to the autonomy of medical doctors in documented or exchanges between the government and the medical profession in the context of reforms.
Change	A transition either induced, contemplated during, or following a reform that has a significant impact from the reformers or the medical profession's standpoint.	Identify differences in pre and post reform conditions. Empirically documented changes highlighting elements of a reform impacting medical doctors. Assessment of the impact of these variations for the medical profession's role, practices, status and autonomy.
Coercion	Change imposed on the medical profession as a consequence of a reform.	Identify situations where the government imposes a policy option without giving the medical profession an opportunity to negotiate or avoid a policy adjustment.
Compliance	Voluntary or non-voluntary adherence to a prescription within the context of reforms.	Situation of adoption by the medical profession of the content of reform (policy, rules, regulations etc).
Compromise	An agreement or settlement between the government and the medical profession that result from concessions.	Identification of the government's and medical doctor's position on the content or process of reforms. Assessment of change in reform as a result of diverging positions and demands from both parties.
Contestation	Strategy to formally oppose components of reforms that may involve political, economic or legal tools such as litigation, strikes, advertising campaigns, etc. More broadly, it is an overt opposition of the medical profession to policy reforms.	Identification of overt opposition by the medical profession through various strategies within each phase of reforms.
Context	Generic and generative concept including the social, legal, political, organisational and economical dimensions that intersect or may intersect with the development and unfolding of reforms. Elements of context can either be distal or proximal (see Chapter 1).	Identify arguments exposing the rational or motives behind a reform. Identify events or situations in the distal or proximal context that precipitated or shaped the content and trajectory of a reform.

(continued)

Constructs and concepts	Definition	Empirical assessment
Influence/power	Generic and generative concept that looks at the capacity to impact the evolution and development of a reform, or on the behaviour of an individual, a group or a circumstance or the effect itself. Manifestations of influence and power are multifaceted.	Identify manifestations of influence or power by the medical profession or the government on a reform (for example, active and successful contestation by medical doctors of productivity targets etc). Identify the adoption of a reform by the government in spite of resistance and opposition from the medical profession. Identifying the inclusion or exclusion within the reform's process of sensitive elements for the medical profession will also be considered as an empirical marker of influence and power.
Interdependence	Varying level of dependence between individuals, tasks or groups with the objective of achieving a common goal.	Identify statements and situations where the need for cooperation between the medical doctors and the government is recognised or factual. Identify elements of sustained collaboration between medical doctors and the government over time in spite of disagreements or divergence.
Leadership	Action of leading a group, an organisation or a project.	Identify individuals taking on a leadership role within government or the medical profession during reforms. Leadership within reforms should manifest itself collectively and in a distributed phenomenon.
Medical profession	Organised bodies representing the interests of medical doctors and the profession within the context of a reform.	Identify groups, associations and organisations within the medical profession that play a role during each phase of the reform.
Negotiated and mediated space	Generic and generative concept that encompasses the interactive field emerging from relationships between governments and the medical profession within the context of a reform.	Empirical assessment of exchanges, negotiations and involvement of actors influencing the development and trajectory of a reform.
Negotiation	An informal and formal process between the medical profession and the government to define a policy that is consequential for reformers or the medical profession.	Identify situations of goal-driven exchanges between the government and the medical profession within a reform with the aim of developing satisfying policies for both parties.

Constructs and concepts	Definition	Empirical assessment
Policy (including policy cycle and instrument)	'Course of action or inaction chosen by public authorities to address a given problem or interrelated set of problems' (Pal, 2006: 2). Reforms consist of a package of policies.	Identify policies that have implications for the role, practice, status and legitimacy of the medical profession.
Politics	Elements of distal and proximal context that relate to parliamentary politics, partisan politics with its own rules and priorities.	Identify situations of political shift in government following an election or political crisis. Also encompasses the political colours of the government in power during a reformative period.
Professionalism	Core values and interest shared by a professional group that may be explicitly introduced in a code of conduct. In our research, it also serves as a heuristic to interpret the voice of the medical profession.	Identify elements that relate to the predispositions of medical doctors and the rational provided by medical doctors to justify their involvement and reactions in the reform.
Proposed reform	Proposed policies, contracts, regulations and accountability mechanisms, part of the reformative process.	Identify content and process for each phase, as formulated by the government in the initial reform project.
Regulation	1) Elaboration or modification of norms in order to control or influence people's behaviours and interactions in healthcare; or 2) The act or process of controlling by rule or restriction; or 3) A rule or order having legal force.	Identifiable regulations proposed or adopted within the context of reforms. Regulations can be identified through the government's attention and reliance on various types of policy instruments or through the valorisation of various norms in discourses.
Relations	Interactions between the government and the medical profession within the negotiated and mediated space.	Identify interactions within the negotiated and mediated space that can be characterised as collaborative or confrontational, intense or sporadic. The characterisation of a relation can be linked to a specific phase of reform and/or around a specific policy option. Relations may also define a confrontational or collaborative trend across periods of reforms.

(continued)

Constructs and concepts	Definition	Empirical assessment
Status legitimacy	1) Lawful status of a government (or governmental actor), a profession or an organisation for the execution of a specific set of tasks; or 2) Publicly recognised status of a government (or governmental actor), a profession, an entity or a group for the execution of a specific set of tasks.	Identify legal substrate of government and medical doctor legitimacy. Identify the consequences of strategies used by the government and medical doctors within the negotiated and mediated space impacting their legitimacy.
Strategies	Course of actions developed by the medical profession or government-reformers to influence the development, unfolding and outcome of reforms.	Identify actions developed by the government or the medical profession to influence the content and process of reform.

References

Abbott, A. (1988) *The System of Professions: An Essay on the Expert Division of Labor*, Chicago, IL: University of Chicago Press.

Abbott, A. (2005) 'Linked ecologies: States and universities as environments for professions', *Sociological Theory*, 23(3): 245–74.

Abel, A.L. and Lewin, W. (1959) 'Report on hospital building', *BMJ*, 1(suppl): 108–14.

Abel-Smith, B. (1964) *The Hospitals, 1800–1948: A Study in Social Administration in England and Wales*, London: Heinemann.

Abramovitz, M. (2005) 'The largely untold story of welfare reform and the human services', *Social Work*, 50(2): 175–86.

Ackroyd, S. (2016) 'Sociological and organisational theories of professions and professionalism', in M. Dent, I. Bourgeault, J.-L. Denis and E. Kuhlman (eds) *The Routledge Companion to the Professions and Professionalism*, Abingdon: Routledge, pp 33–48.

Ackroyd, S., Hughes, J. and Soothill, K. (1989) 'Public sector services and their management', *Journal of Management Studies*, 26(6): 603–19.

ACMDPQ (Association des conseils des médecins, dentistes et pharmaciens du Québec) (2014) 'Mémoire de l'Association des conseils des médecins, dentistes et pharmaciens du Québec', Projet de loi n° 10: Loi modifiant l'organisation et la gouvernance du réseau de la santé et des services sociaux notamment par l'abolition des agences régionales, présenté à la Commission de la santé et des services sociaux, novembre.

Adams, T.L. (2015) 'Sociology of professions: International divergences and research directions', *Work, Employment and Society*, 29(1): 154–65.

Adler, P.S. and Kwon, S.W. (2013) 'The mutation of professionalism as a contested diffusion process: Clinical guidelines as carriers of institutional change in medicine', *Journal of Management Studies*, 50(5): 930–62.

Adler, P.S., Kwon, S.W. and Heckscher, C. (2008) 'Perspective – Professional work: The emergence of collaborative community', *Organization Science*, 19(2): 359–76.

Adler, P.S., Heckscher, C., McCarthy, J.E. and Rubinstein, S.A. (2015) 'The mutations of professional responsibility: Toward collaborative community', in D.E. Mitchell and R.K. Ream (eds) *Professional Responsibility*, Cham: Springer, pp 309–26.

Aggarwal, M. (2009) 'Primary care reform: A case study of Ontario', Doctoral dissertation, Doctor of Philosophy, Department of Health Policy, Management and Evaluation, University of Toronto.

Ahmed, H., Brown, A. and Saks, M. (2018) 'Patterns of medical oversight and regulation in Canada', in J.M. Chamberlain, M. Dent and M. Saks (eds) *Professional Health Regulation in the Public Interest: International Perspectives*, Bristol: Policy Press, pp 135–59.

AJMQ (Association des jeunes médecins du Québec) (1998) 'Mémoire de l'Association des jeunes médecins du Québec concernant le projet de loi n°404, loi modifiant la loi sur les services sociaux et modifiant diverses dispositions législatives', 24 février.

Alam, N. (2016) 'Why I'm voting "no"', *Medical Post*, 52(9).

Alford, R.R. (1977) *Health Care Politics: Ideological and Interest Group Barriers to Reform*, Chicago, IL: University of Chicago Press.

Allen, U.D., Collins, T., Sefa Dei, G.J., Henry, F., Ibrahim, A. and James, C.E. (2021) *Impacts of COVID-19 in Racialized Communities*, Ottawa: Royal Society of Canada.

Alvarez-Rosete, A. and Mays, N. (2008) 'Reconciling two conflicting tales of the English health policy process since 1997', *British Politics*, 3: 183–2.

Alvarez-Rosete, A. and Mays, N. (2014) 'Understanding NHS policy making in England: The formulation of the NHS plan 2000', *The British Journal of Politics and International Relations*, 16: 624–44.

AMQ (Association médicale du Québec) (2017) 'Cohérence et régulation dans l'organisation clinique et dans la gestion des établissements: Misons sur le partenariat médico-administratif', Mémoire de l'Association médicale du Québec, Projet de loi n°130, Loi modifiant certaines dispositions relatives à l'organisation clinique et à la gestion des établissements de santé et de services sociaux, février.

AMQ and CMA (Canadian Medical Association) (2015) 'Accessibilité: La solution passe par la concertation', Mémoire conjoint de l'Association médicale du Québec et de l'Association médicale canadienne, Projet de loi no 20: Loi édictant la Loi favorisant l'accès aux services de médecine de famille et de médecine spécialisée et modifiant diverses dispositions législatives en matière de procréation assistée, 25 mars.

Anonymous (2016) 'Why I'm voting "yes"', *Medical Post*, 52(9): 9.

Ansell, C. and Gash, A. (2008) 'Collaborative governance in theory and practice', *Journal of Public Administration Research & Theory*, 18: 543–71.

Association pour l'accès à l'avortement c. Québec, 2006 QCCS 4694, [2006] RJQ 1938t

Baggott, R. (2015) *Understanding Health Policy*, Bristol: Policy Press.

Baker, G.R. and Denis, J.L. (2011) 'Medical leadership in health care systems: From professional authority to organizational leadership', *Public Money & Management*, 31(5): 355–62.

Baker, G.R., Norton, P.G., Flintoft, V., Blais, R., Brown, A., Cox, J. et al (2004) 'The Canadian Adverse Events Study: The incidence of adverse events among hospital patients in Canada', *Canadian Medical Association Journal*, 170(11): 1678–86.

Barnard, K. and Lee, K. (1977) *Conflicts in the National Health Service*, London: Croom Helm.

Barnett, H. (2020) *Constitutional and Administrative Law*, Abingdon: Routledge.

Barry, N.P. (1989) *An Introduction to Modern Political Theory* (2nd edn), Basingstoke: Macmillan.

BCMA (British Columbia Medical Association) (2000) *Turning the Tide – Saving Medicare for Canadians, Part I of II Laying the Foundation for Sustaining Medicare*, A Discussion Paper by BC's Physicians, July.

Beaulieu, C. (1987) 'Un conseil exécutoire de médiation pourra réduire les horaires de travail des internes', *Le Devoir*, 19 novembre.

Bejerot, E. and Hasselbladh, H. (2011) 'Professional autonomy and pastoral power: The transformation of quality registers in Swedish health care', *Public Administration*, 89(4): 1604–21.

Bélanger, J.-P. (1992) 'De la Commission Castonguay à la Commission Rochon ... Vingt ans d'histoire de l'évolution des services de santé et des services sociaux au Québec', *Service Social*, 41(2): 49–70.

Belluz, J. (2012a) 'The new doctor war: Are MDs losing bargaining power?', *Medical Post*, 48(10) 8, 10.

Belluz, J. (2012b) 'OMA board recommends "yes" vote to new fee deal', *Medical Post*, 48(20) 10.

Belluz, J. (2012c) 'Ontario LHINs to oversee primary care: Minister', *Medical Post*, 48(3) 6.

Besly, N., Goldsmith, T., Rogers, R. and Walters, R.H. (2018) *How Parliament Works*, London: Taylor & Francis.

Beveridge, W.H. (1942) *Social Insurance and Allied Services*, London: HMO.

Bevir, M. (2010) 'Rethinking governmentality: Towards genealogies of governance', *European Journal of Social Theory*, 13(4): 423–41.

Bevir, M. (2011) 'Governance and governmentality after neoliberalism', *Policy & Politics*, 39(4): 457–71.

Bevir, M. (2013) *A Theory of Governance*, University of California, e-Scholarship.

Bevir, M. and Waring, J. (2018) *Decentring Health Policy: Learning from British Experiences in Healthcare Governance*, Abingdon: Routledge.

Bevir, M., Rhodes, R.A. and Weller, P. (2003) 'Comparative governance: Prospects and lessons', *Public Administration*, 81(1): 191–210.

Bhatia, R.S., Chu, C., Pang, A., Tadrous, M., Stamenova, V. and Cram, P. (2021) 'Virtual care use before and during the COVID-19 pandemic: A repeated cross-sectional study', *CMAJ Open*, 9(1): E107.

Blanchet, N.J. and Fox, A.M. (2013) 'Prospective political analysis for policy design: Enhancing the political viability of single-payer health reform in Vermont', *Health Policy*, 111: 78–85.

Blau, P. and Scott, W.R. (1962) *Formal Organizations*, San Francisco, CA: Chandler.

Bloomfield, B. and Best, A. (1992) 'Management consultants, systems development, power and the translation of problems', *The Sociological Review*, 40(3): 533–60.

British Medical Association (BMA) (1942) *Medical Planning Commission: Draft Interim Report*, London: BMA.

BMA (1969) *Health Services Financing*, London: BMA.

BMA (2010) *Equity and Excellence: Liberating the NHS – BMA Response*, London: BMA.

BMA (2015) *Junior Doctors: Contract Proposals for Junior Doctors*, London: BMA.

BMA (2020) *COVID-19: Ethical Issues – A Guidance Note*. Available at: www.bma.org.uk/media/2360/bma-covid-19-ethics-guidance-april-2020.pdf

BMA (2021) *Member Briefing: Government Health White Paper*, London: BMA.

British Medical Journal (BMJ) (1950) 'A falling policy', 2: 1262–3.

BMJ (1963) 'Discontent with-', 2: 1143–4.

BMJ (1964) 'The basis of unity', 1: 253–4.

BMJ (1969) 'On the brink', 5640: 329.

BMJ (1972) 'Sir Paul Chambers: Report of an inquiry into the association's constitution and organization', 2: 45–67.

BMJ (1974) 'Damaging and needles collision', 4: 305–6.

BMJ (1975) 'Report of the proceedings of the Central Committee for Hospital Medicine Services', 4: 593–5.

BMJ (1977) 'Discussion document on ethical responsibilities of doctors practising in the national health service', 1: 157–9.

BMJ (1978) 'The disalienation of the NHS', 2: 12.

BMJ (1980) 'New NHS structure needs new attitudes', 281: 342–2.

BMJ (1983) 'Business management for the NHS?', 287: 1321–2.

BMJ (1985) 'Gridlock and incentives in NHS', 291: 992–3.

BMJ (1986) 'BMA's statement', 292: 1152.

BMJ (1988) 'Evidence to the government internal review of the national health service', 296: 1411–13.

BMJ (1989) 'BMA launches campaign against white paper', 298: 676–9.

Borsellino, M. (1998a) 'OMA snap election', *Medical Post*, 34(2): 2.

Borsellino, M. (1998b) 'Pilot sites chosen for Ontario primary care project', *Medical Post*, 34(21): 12.

Borsellino, M. (2000) 'Ontario NPs seeking their place', *Medical Post*, 36(33): 51.

Borsellino, M. (2003) 'Bill 8 not great, say Ont MDs', *Medical Post*, 39(46): 1.

Borsellino, M. (2004a) 'Ontario doctors blast medicare legislation', *Medical Post*, 40(10): 2.

Borsellino, M. (2004b) 'OMA lobbying effects amendments to Bill 8', *Medical Post*, 40(14): 9.

Borsellino, M. (2004c) 'Ontario doctors mull over complex package', *Medical Post*, 40(37): 1.

Borsellino, M. (2004d) 'Ont. deal a no-go?', *Medical Post*, 40(42): 1.

Borsellino, M. (2004e) 'Imposing contract', *Medical Post*, 40(47): 2.

Borsellino, M. (2005a) 'Ontario's 11% solution', *Medical Post*, 41(11): 1.

Borsellino, M. (2005b) 'One unexpected result of the OMA agreement', *Medical Post*, 41(14): 12.

Borsellino, M. (2005c) 'New president turns attention to wait times, disease prevention', *Medical Post*, 41(20): 27.

Borsellino, M. (2005d) 'Ontario's wait-time czar offers answers', *Medical Post*, 41(23): 23.

Borsellino, M. (2005e) 'Winning the waiting game', *Medical Post*, 41(22): 31.

Borsellino, M. (2010a) 'Hospital prototype bylaws draw MD's fire', *Medical Post*, 46(10): 41.

Borsellino, M. (2010b) 'Money at root of OMA/OHA battle', *Medical Post*, 46(8): 8.

Bourque, M. and Leruste, G. (2010) 'La transformation des idées sur la privatisation du système de santé québécois depuis 1970: Le passage à un nouveau référentiel sectoriel?', *Politique et sociétés*, 29(2): 105–29.

Boutrouille, L., Régis, C. and Pomey, M.-P. (2021) 'Enjeux juridiques propres au modèle émergent des patients accompagnateurs dans les milieux de soins au Québec', Revue juridique, Thémis de l'université de Montréal, 55–1.

Boylan-Kemp, J. (ed) (2008) *The English Legal System – The Fundamentals*, London: Sweet & Maxwell.

Boyle, T. (2016a) 'MDs battle each other in contract vote', *Toronto Star*, 14 August.

Boyle, T. (2016b) 'Doctors association could turn into union', *Toronto Star*, 26 August.

Boyle, T. (2017a) 'MDs vote on ousting OMA heads', *Toronto Star*, 28 January.

Boyle, T. (2017b) 'OMA executive committee resigns', *Toronto Star*, 7 February.

Bradburn, J. (2018) 'In the mood for cuts: How the "Common Sense Revolution" swept Ontario in 1995', *TVO*, 8 June. Available at: www.tvo.org/article/in-the-mood-for-cuts-how-the-common-sense-revolution-swept-ontario-in-1995

Braverman, H. (1974) *Labor and Monopoly Capital*, New York, NY: Monthly Review Press.

Breton, P. and Sirois, A. (2002) 'Guerre ouverte avec Québec', *La Presse*, 1 novembre.

Brint, S. (1993) 'Eliot Freidson's contribution to the sociology of professions', *Work and Occupations*, 20(3): 259–78.

Brock, D.M., Powell, M.J. and Hinings, C. (2007) 'Archetypal change and the professional service firm', in A.B. Shani and D.A. Noumair (eds) *Research in Organizational Change and Development*, Kidlington: Emerald Group Publishing Limited, pp 221–51.

Brock, D.M., Leblebici, H. and Muzio, D. (2013) 'Understanding professionals and their workplaces: The mission of the *Journal of Professions and Organization*', *Journal of Professions and Organization*, 1(1): 1–15.

Bronca, T. (2015) 'The high cost of care', *Medical Post*, 51(2): 19–23.

Bronca, T. (2016a) 'Hundreds of doctors endorse five principles to guide future negotiations', *Medical Post*, 52(11): 10.

Bronca, T. (2016b) 'Concerned Ontario doctors: Putting faces on the cuts', *Medical Post*, 52(6): 10.

Bronca, T. (2016c) 'Turmoil hits Ontario doctor groups after fee deal voted down', *Medical Post*, 52(10) 13–14.

Bronca, T. (2016d) 'Hundreds of doctors endorse five principles to guide future negotiations', *Medical Post*, 52(11): 10.

Bronca, T. (2019) 'The specialists' divorce', *Medical Post*.

Brown, P. and Flores, R. (2018) 'The informalisation of professional–patient interactions and the consequences for regulation in the United Kingdom', in J.M. Chamberlain, M. Dent and M. Saks (eds) *Professional Health Regulation in the Public Interest: International Perspectives*, Bristol: Policy Press, pp 39–59.

Buchanan, B. (1974) 'Building organizational commitment: The socialization of managers in work organizations', *Administrative Science Quarterly*, 19: 509–32.

Calnan, M. and Gabe, J. (1991) 'Recent developments in general practice: A sociological analysis', in M. Calnan, J. Gabe and M. Bury (eds) *The Sociology of the Health Service*, Abingdon: Routledge, pp 150–71.

Cameron, J. (1965) *A Charter for the Family Doctor Service*, London: BMA.

Campbell, A.L. (2011) 'Policy feedbacks and the impact of policy designs on public opinion', *Journal of Health Politics, Policy, and Law*, 36(6): 961–73.

Campbell, C. (2009) 'Distinguishing the power of agency from agentic power: A note on Weber and the "black box" of personal agency', *Sociological Theory*, 27(4): 407–18.

Campbell, D. (2010) 'Doctors warned to expect unrest over NHS reforms', *The Guardian*, 19 November.

Campbell, D. (2015) 'Junior doctors likely to strike as government talks falter', *The Guardian*, 29 December.

Carpenter, D. (2012) 'Is health politics different?', *Annual Review of Political Science*, 15: 287–311.

Cary, P. (2005) 'Process under scrutiny', *Medical Post*, 41(10): 13.

Central Committee for Hospital Medical Services (1988) *NHS Funding: The Crisis in the Acute Hospital Sector*, London: BMA.

Central Health Services Council (1954) *Report of the Committee on General Practice within the National Health Service* (Cohen Committee), London: HMSO.

Chalvin, S. (1971) 'Hôpitaux et médecins s'élèvent contre la réorganisation projetée', *Le Devoir*, 6 octobre.

Chamberlain, J.M., Dent, M. and Saks, M. (eds) (2018) *Professional Health Regulation in the Public Interest: International Perspectives*, Bristol: Policy Press.

Chaoulli vs Québec (Attorney General), 2005 SCC 35 (CanLII), [2005] 1 SCR 791.

Chief Medical Officer (2006) *Good Doctors, Safer Patients*, London: Department of Health.

Chouinard, T. (2016) 'Nouvelle collision entre Barrette et les fédérations de médecins', *La Presse*, 10 decembre.

Clarke, M. and Stewart, J. (1997) *Handling the Wicked Issues – A Challenge for Government*, Birmingham: University of Birmingham.

Clegg, S.R. (1989) *Frameworks of Power*, London: SAGE Publications Ltd.

Cloutier, C., Denis, J.L., Langley, A., and Lamothe, L. (2016) 'Agency at the managerial interface: Public sector reform as institutional work', *Journal of Public Administration Research and Theory*, 26(2): 259–76.

CMA (Canadian Medical Association) (1976) 'Ontario Health Ministry prepares plans to close 3000 hospital beds, save $50 million', *Canadian Medical Association Journal*, 144: 455.

CMA (1984) 'OMA to challenge Canada Health Act in the courts', *Canadian Medical Association Journal*, 131(2): 125–8.

CMA (1993) 'OHIP holds back 4.8% of payments to MDs', *Canadian Medical Association Journal*, 149(10): 1499.

CMA (2010) *Health Care Transformation in Canada: Change that Works, Care that Lasts*. Available at: http://policybase.cma.ca/dbtw-wpd/PolicyPDF/PD10-05.PDF

CMA (2021) *COVID-19 Long-Term Considerations for the Canadian Medical Association*, Ottawa.

Collège des medecins du Québec (CMQ) (2005) 'Mémoire du Collège des medecins du Québec: Projet de loi n°83', Loi modifiant la Loi sur les services de santé et les services sociaux et d'autres dispositions législatifves, présenté à la Commission des affaires sociales, 21 janvier.

CMQ (College of Physicians of Quebec) (2014) 'Projet de loi n°10: Loi modifiant l'organisation et la gouvernance du réseau de la santé et des services sociaux notamment par l'abolition des agences régionales', Mémoire présenté à la Commission de la santé et des services sociaux, CSSS – 006M CP – PL 10 Abolition des agences régionales, Collège des médecins du Québec, 20 octobre.

CMQ (2017) 'Mémoire Projet de loi n°130, Loi modifiant certaines dispositions relatives à l'organisation clinique et à la gestion des établissements de santé et de services sociaux', Mémoire présenté à la Commission de la santé et des services sociaux, 7 février.

Coburn, D. (1993) 'State authority, medical dominance, and trends in the regulation of the health professions: The Ontario case', *Social Science & Medicine*, 37(2): 129.

Coburn, D., Rappolt, S. and Bourgeault, I. (1997) 'Decline vs retention of medical power through restratification: An examination of the Ontario Case', *Sociology of Health & Illness*, 19(1): 1–22.

Collins, R. and Sanderson, S.K. (2015) *Conflict Sociology: A Sociological Classic Updated*, Abingdon: Routledge.

Commission d'enquête sur les services de santé et les services sociaux, Rochon, J. (Commissaire) (1988) *Rapport de la Commission d'enquête sur les services de santé et les services sociaux*, Québec: Publications du Québec.

Commission d'enquête sur la santé et le bien-être social – Québec, C. Castonguay et G. Nepveu (Commissaires) (1967–72) *Rapport de la Commission d'enquête sur la santé et le bien-être social*, Québec: Éditeur officiel du Québec.

Commission d'étude sur les services de santé et les services sociaux – Québec, M. Clair (Commissaire) (2000) *Rapport et recommandations – Les solutions émergentes*, Québec: Publications du Québec.

Commission de la santé (1969) *Journal des débats*, Commission des sciences de la santé B-2181, Commission de la santé, Fascicule no 36, 22 mai.

Commission permanente des affaires sociales (1971) Projet de loi no 65, Loi de l'organisation des services de santé et des services sociaux, Journal des débats de la Commission permanente des affaires sociales, 5 octobre, 11(88).

Constitution Acts (1867–82) Constitution Act, 1867, 30 and 31 Victoria, c. 3 (UK) An Act for the Union of Canada, Nova Scotia, and New Brunswick, and the Government thereof; and for Purposes connected therewith, 29 March 1867. Available at: https://laws-lois.justice.gc.ca/eng/const/page-1.html

Contandriopoulos, A.P., Lemay, A., Tessier, G. and Champagne, F. (1989) 'Modalités de financement et contrôle des coûts du système de soins: l'exemple du Québec', *Sciences sociales et santé*, 7(4): 113–37.

Cooper, D.J. and Robson, K. (2006) 'Accounting, professions and regulation: Locating the sites of professionalization', *Accounting, Organizations and Society*, 31: 415–44.

Courpasson, D., Dany, F. and Clegg, S. (2012) 'Resisters at work: Generating productive resistance in the workplace', *Organization Science*, 23(3): 801–19.

CPHA (Canadian Public Health Association) (1995) 'Le transfert canadien en matière de santé et des programmes sociaux et l'équité en matière de santé'. Available at: www.cpha.ca/fr/le-transfert-canadien-en-matiere-de-sante-et-des-programmes-sociaux-et-lequite-en-matiere-de-sante

CPSO (College of Physicians and Surgeons of Ontario) (2009) The College of Physicians and Surgeons of Ontario's Submission on Bill 179 – The Regulated Health Professions Statute Law Amendment Act, 2009, 25 September, 18.

Crane, R.T. (1907) *State in Constitutional and International Law*, Baltimore, MD: Johns Hopkins Press.

Crawford, T. (1984) 'Norton won't rule out extra-billing ban', *Toronto Star*, 2 August.

Crinson, I. (1998) 'Putting patients first: The continuity of the consumerist discourse in health policy, from radical right to New Labour', *Critical Social Policy*, 18(55): 227–39.

Crinson, I. (2009) *Health Policy: A Critical Perspective*, London: SAGE Publications Ltd.

Crompton, R. (1990) 'Professions in the current context', *Work, Employment and Society*, 4(5): 147–66.

Crowe, P. (1982) 'Family OHIP could go up by $10', *Toronto Star*, 4 May.

Cruess, R.L., Cruess, S.R. and Johnston, S.E. (2000) 'Professionalism: An ideal to be sustained', *The Lancet*, 356(9224): 156–9.

Cruess, S.R., Johnston, S. and Cruess, R.L. (2004) ' "Profession": A working definition for medical educators', *Teaching and Learning in Medicine*, 16(1): 74–6.

Cruickshank, G. and Jenkins, A. (2014) 'Re: NHS England's five year plan', *British Medical Journal*, 349: g6484.

Dacin, T.M., Goodstein, J. and Scott, R.W. (2002) 'Institutional theory and institutional change: Introduction to the special research forum', *Academy of Management Journal*, 45(1): 45–56.

Daoust, G. (1971) 'Les omnipraticiens veulent un rôle de participation', *La Presse*, 6 octobre.

Daoust-Boivert, A. (2014a) 'Étalement: Les spécialistes disent oui', *Le Devoir*, 27 septembre.

Daoust-Boivert, A. (2014b) 'Les critiques s'accumulent', *Le Devoir*, 23 octobre.

Dawson, S. and Dargie, C. (2002) 'New public management: A discussion with special reference to UK health', in K. McLaughlin, S.P. Osborne and E. Ferlie (eds) *New Public Management: Current Trends and Future Prospects*, London: Routledge, pp 34–56.

Day, P. and Klein, R. (1985) 'Central accountability and local decision making: Towards a new NHS', *British Medical Journal*, 290: 1676.

Day, P. and Klein, R. (1991) 'Britain's health care experiment', *Health Affairs*, 10: 39–59.

Day, P. and Klein, R. (1992) 'Constitutional and distributional conflict in British medical politics: The case of general practice, 1911–1991', *Political Studies*, 40: 462–78.

De Bruijn, J.A. (2010) *Managing Professionals*, London: Routledge.

deCarteret Cory, P. (2005) 'Study, conclusions and recommendations pertaining to medical audit practice in Ontario', 21 April, 326.

Demers, L. (2003) 'La profession médicale et l'État: Le système de santé au Québec – Organisations, acteurs, enjeux', in V. Lemieux, P. Bergeron, C. Bégin and G. Bélanger (eds) *Le système de santé au Québec*, Québec: Presses de l'Université Laval, pp 261–96.

Demont, J. (2003) 'Liberals win Ontario 2003 election', *The Canadian Encyclopedia*, 25 November.

Denhardt, R.B. and Denhardt, J.V. (2000) 'The new public service: Serving rather than steering', *Public Administration Review*, 60(6): 549–59.

Denis, J. -L. and van Gestel, N. (2016) 'Medical doctors in healthcare leadership: Theoretical and practical challenges', *BMC Health Services Research*, 16(2): 158.

Denis, J.-L., Langley, A. and Rouleau, L. (2006) 'The power of numbers in strategizing', *Strategic Organization*, 4(4): 349–77.

Denis, J.-L., Baker, G.R., Black, C., Langley, A., Lawless, B., Leblanc, D. et al (2013) *Exploring the Dynamics of Physician Engagement and Leadership for Health System Improvement: Prospects for Canadian Healthcare Systems*, Report on physician engagement and leadership for health system improvement, CIHR/ CFHI.

Denis, J.-L., van Gestel, N. and Lepage, A. (2016) 'Professional agency, leadership and organizational change', in M. Dent, I.L. Bourgeault, J-L. Denis and E. Kuhlmann (eds) *The Routledge Companion to the Professions and Professionalism*, Abingdon: Routledge, pp 215–27.

Denis, J.-L., Côté, N., Fleury, C., Currie, G. and Spyridonidis, D. (2021) 'Global health and innovation: A panoramic view on health human resources in the COVID-19 pandemic context', *The International Journal of Health Planning and Management*, 36(S1): 58–70.

Denning, M., Goh, E.T., Tan, B., Kanneganti, A., Almonte, M., Scott, A. et al (2021) 'Determinants of burnout and other aspects of psychological well-being in healthcare workers during the Covid-19 pandemic: A multinational cross-sectional study', *PLoS One*, 16(4): e0238666. Available at: https://doi.org/10.1371/journal.pone.0238666

Dent, M. (2018) 'Health care governance, user involvement and medical regulation in Europe', in J.M. Chamberlain, M. Dent and M. Saks (eds) *Professional Health Regulation in the Public Interest: International Perspectives*, Bristol: Policy Press, pp 17–37.

Department of Health and Social Care (2021) *Integration and Innovation: Working Together to Improve Health and Social Care*, London: The Stationery Office.

des Rivières, P. (1982) 'Selon le CPQ, Québec aurait tort de geler unilatéralement les salaires', *Le Devoir*, 14 mai.

Desrosiers, G. (1986) 'The Québec health care system', *Journal of Public Health Policy*, 7(2): 211–17.

Deverell, J. (1986) 'Doctors stand alone on extra billing', *Toronto Star*, 17 January.

DH (Department of Health) (2001) *Shifting the Balance of Power within the NHS – Securing Delivery*, London: DH.

DHSS (Department of Health and Social Services) (1971) *National Health Service Reorganisation: Consultative Document*, London: HMSO.

DHSS (1979) *Patients first: Consultative paper on the structure and management of the National Health Service in England and Wales*, London, HMSO.

DHSS (1983) *NHS Management Inquiry* (Griffiths Report), London: HMSO.

Dickinson, H., Bismark, M., Phelps, G. and Loh, E. (2016) 'Future of medical engagement', *Australian Health Review*, 40(4): 443–6.

DiMaggio, P.J. and Powell, W.W. (1983) 'The iron cage revisited: Institutional isomorphism and collective rationality in organizational fields', *American Sociological Review*, 48: 147–60.

DiMaggio, P.J. and Powell, W.W. (1991) *The New Institutionalism in Organizational Analysis*, Chicago, IL: University of Chicago Press.

Dingwall, R. (2016) *Essays on Professions*, Abingdon: Routledge.

Dixon, J. and Dewar, S. (2000) 'The NHS plan: As good as it gets – make the most of it', *British Medical Journal*, 321: 315–16.

Dobrow, M.J., Goel V., Lemieux-Charles, L. and Black, N.A. (2006) 'The impact of context on evidence utilization: A framework for expert groups developing health policy recommendations', *Social Science & Medicine*, 63(7): 1811–24.

Doern, G.B. and Phidd, R.W. (1992) *Canadian Public Policy: Ideas, Structure, Process* (2nd edn), Toronto, ON: Nelson.

Doig, J. (1967) 'OMSIP cheques shredded, NDP says', *Toronto Star*, 3 May.

Dowling, B. (2000) *GPs and Purchasing in the NHS: The Internal Market and Beyond*, Aldershot: Ashgate Publishing Limited.

Drazin, R. (1990) 'Professionals and innovation: Structural-functional versus radical-structural perspectives', *Journal of Management Studies*, 27(3): 245–63.

Drummond, D. (2012) *Public Services for Ontarians: A Path to Sustainability and Excellence*, Commission on the Reform of Ontario's Public Services, Queen's Printer for Ontario. Available at: www.fin.gov.on.ca/en/reformcommission

Dunlop, M. (1971) 'Doctors are warned they're losing right to determine income', *Toronto Star*, 10 August.

Dunlop, M. (1972a) 'Doctors may help set up health centres', *Toronto Star*, 26 August.

Dunlop, M. (1972b) 'Looking after healthy waster of money: MDs', *Toronto Star*, 25 September.

Dunlop, M. (1980) 'Doctors seek better deal from OHIP', *Toronto Star*, 7 June.

Dunlop, M. and Newbery, L. (1985) 'MDs vow all-out battle against "dictatorial" bill', *Toronto Star*, 21 December.

Dupre, M. (1970) 'Québec ne pliera pas au chantage des professionnels de la santé', *La Presse*, 4 juillet.

Dussault, G. (1975) 'Les médecins du Québec (1940–1970)', *Recherches sociographiques*, 16(1): 69–84.

Dutrisac, C. (1970a) 'Les médecins spécialistes: Non au projet de loi de Castonguay', *La Presse*, 3 juillet.

Dutrisac, C. (1970b) 'Assurance-maladie. Les médecins veulent pouvoir se soustraire à l'entente de la Fédération avec Québec', *La Presse*, 7 juillet.

Dyer, C. (2001) 'Bristol inquiry condemns hospital's club "culture"', *British Medical Journal*, 323: 181.

Eckstein, H. (1958) *The English Health Service: Its Origins, Structure, and Achievements*, Cambridge, MA: Harvard University Press.

Eckstein, H. (1960) *Pressure Group Politics: The Case of the British Medical Association*, Redwood City, CA: Stanford University Press.

Elliott, O.V. and Salamon, L.M. (2002) *The Tools of Government: A Guide to the New Governance*, Oxford: Oxford University Press.

Elshaug, A.G., Rosenthal, M.B., Lavis, J.N., Brownlee, S., Schmidt, H., Nagpal, S. et al (2017) 'Levers for addressing medical underuse and overuse: Achieving high-value health care', *The Lancet*, 390(10090): 191–202.

Elston, M.A. (2002) 'The politics of professional power: Medicine in a changing health service', in M. Bury, M. Calnan and J. Gabe (eds) *The Sociology of the Health Service*, Abingdon: Routledge, pp 68–98.

Emirbayer, M. and Mische, A. (1998) 'What is agency?', *American Journal of Sociology*, 103(4): 962–1023.

Estabrooks, C.A., Straus, S.E., Flood, C. M., Keefe, J., Armstrong, P., Donner, G.J. et al (2020) *Restoring Trust: COVID-19 and the Future of Long-Term Care in Canada*, Ottawa, ON: Royal Society of Canada.

Etzioni, A. (1969) *The Semi-Professions and Their Organization: Teachers, Nurses, Social Workers*, New York, NY: Free Press.

Evetts, J. (2004) 'Organizational or occupational professionalism: Centralized regulation or occupational trust', Paper presented at the ISA RC52 Interim Conference, Versailles, France.

Evetts, J. (2011) 'A new professionalism? Challenges and opportunities', *Current Sociology*, 59(4): 406–22.

Evetts, J. (2013) 'Professionalism: Value and ideology', *Current Sociology*, 61(5–6): 778–96.

Expenditure Committee (1971) Employment and Social Services Sub-Committee, Minutes of Evidence, 31 March 1971, Session 1970–1, HC 323ii, London: HMSO.

Exworthy, M., Mannion, R. and Martin, P. (2016) *Dismantling the NHS: Evaluating the Impact of Health Reforms*, Bristol: Policy Press.

Facal, J. (2006) *Volonté politique et pouvoir médical. La naissance de l'assurance-maladie au Québec et aux États-Unis*, Montréal, QC: Les Éditions du Boréal.

Ferguson, J. (1986) 'MDs meet to decide job action', *Toronto Star*, 18 January.

Ferguson, R. (1986) 'How doctors wrote wrong prescription for effective strike', *Toronto Star*, 26 July.

Ferlie, E. and McGivern, G. (2013) 'Bringing Anglo-governmentality into public management scholarship: The case of evidence-based medicine in UK health care', *Journal of Public Administration Research and Theory*, 24(1): 59–83.

Ferlie, E., Musselin, C. and Andresani, G. (2008) 'The steering of higher education systems: A public management perspective', *Higher Education*, 56(3): 325.

Ferlie, E., Fitzgerald, L., Wood, M. and Hawkins, C. (2005) 'The nonspread of innovations: The mediating role of professionals', *Academy of Management Journal*, 48: 117–34.

Fiset-Laniel, J., Guyon, A.I., Perreault, R. and Strumpf, E.C. (2020) 'Public health investments: Neglect or wilful omission? Historical trends in Québec and implications for Canada', *Canadian Journal of Public Health*, 111: 383–8.

Fitzgerald, L. and Dopson, S. (2009) 'Comparative case study designs: Their utility and development in organisational research', in D.A. Buchanan and A. Bryman (eds) *The SAGE Handbook of Organizational Research Methods*, London: SAGE Publications Ltd, pp 465–83.

Flavelle, D. (1985) 'Billing ban means war: MDs', *Toronto Star*, 6 July.

Flood, C.M. and Joanna Erdman, J. (2004) 'The boundaries of Medicare: Tensions in the dual role of Ontario's physician services review committee', working paper, 12:1 HLJ1.

Flood, C.M. and Thomas, B. (2016) 'Modernizing the Canada Health Act', *Dalhousie Law Journal*, 39: 397.

FMOQ (Fédération des médecins omnipraticiens du Québec) (1996) 'Mémoire à la Commission parlementaire des affaires sociales relativement au projet de loi 116 modifiant à nouveau la Loi sur les services de santé et les services sociaux', 17 mai.

FMOQ (1998) 'Mémoire à la Commission parlementaire des affaires sociales relativement au projet de loi 404 modifiant à nouveau la Loi sur les services de santé et les services sociaux', 26 février.

FMOQ (2001) 'Mémoire à la Commission parlementaire des affaires sociales relativement au projet de loi n° 28 modifiant à nouveau la Loi sur les services de santé et les services sociaux', 5 juin.

FMOQ (2003) 'Mémoire à la Commission des affaires sociales relativement au projet de loi n° 25, Loi sur les agences de développement de réseaux locaux de services se danté et de services sociaux', 2 décembre.

FMOQ (2005) 'Résumé du Mémoire de la FMOQ à la Commission des affaires sociales relativement au projet de loi n° 83, Loi modifiant la loi sur les services de santé et les services sociaux et d'autres dispositions législatives', Janvier.

FMOQ (2006) 'Mémoire de la Fédération des médecins omnipraticiens du Québec à la Commission des affaires sociales, Projet de loi n° 33, Loi modifiant la loi sur les services de santé et les services sociaux et d'autres dispositions législatives', 13 septembre.

FMOQ (2014) 'Mémoire de la FMOQ présenté à la Commission de la santé et des services sociaux. Concernant le projet de loi n° 10: Loi modifiant l'organisation et la gouvernance du réseau de la santé et des services sociaux notamment par l'abolition des agences régionales', CSSS – 010M CP – PL 10 Abolition des agences régionales, octobre.

FMOQ (2015a) 'Mémoire de la Fédération des médecins omnipraticiens du Québec présenté à la Commission de la santé et des services sociaux. Concernant le projet de loi n°20: Loi édictant la Loi favorisant l'accès aux services de médecine de famille et de médecine spécialisée et modifiant diverses dispositions législatives en matière de procréation assistée', CSSS – 045M, CP – PL 20, Accès services de médecine, mars.

FMOQ (2015b) 'Adoption du projet de loi 20: une loi inutile et contre-productive', Press release, Fédération des médecins omnipraticiens du Québec, 10 novembre.

FMOQ (2017) 'Mémoire de la Fédération des médecins omnipraticiens du Québec (FMOQ) présenté à la Commission de la santé et des services sociaux. Concernant le projet de loi n° 130: Loi modifiant certaines dispositions relatives à l'organisation clinique et à la gestion des établissements de santé et de services sociaux', CSSS – 013M, CP – PL 130, Organisation clinique, fevrier.

FMOQ, FMSQ and FMRQ (2002) 'Crise dans les urgences: les médecins omnipraticiens, spécialistes et résidents', Press release, 11 juillet.

FMRQ (Fédération des médecins résidents du Québec) (1996) 'Commentaires de la Fédération des médecins résidents du Québec sur le projet loi n° 116: Loi modifiant de nouveau la loi sur les services de santé et les services sociaux', Présentés lors des audiences de la Commission parlementaire des affaires sociales, 23 mai.

FMRQ (2001) 'Mémoire concernant le Projet de loi n° 28 modifiant à nouveau la Loi sur les services de santé et les services sociaux et modifiant diverses dispositions législatives', 6 juin.

FMSQ (Fédération des médecins spécialistes du Québec) (1991) *Manifeste: La médecine ligotée: Projet de loi n° 120.*

FMSQ (1996) Lettre à la Commission parlementaire des affaires sociales, 23 mai.

FMSQ (1998) 'Avis Projet de loi 404 pour discussion en Commission parlementaire', 26 février.

FMSQ (2000a) 'Mémoire relatif au financement et à l'organisation des services de santé des services sociaux dans le cadre de la Commission d'étude sur les services de santé et les services sociaux', Présenté par la Fédération des médecins spécialistes du Québec, 21 septembre.

FMSQ (2000b) 'La Fédération des médecins spécialistes du Québec donne son point de vue sur le système public de santé québécois dans le cadre de la Commission Clair', Presse release, 25 octobre.

FMSQ (2001) 'Mémoire de la Fédération des médecins spécialistes du Québec. Projet de loi n° 28: Loi modifiant la Loi sur les services sociaux e modifiant diverses dispositions législatives', Présenté à la Commission parlementaire des affaires sociales, 6 juin.

FMSQ (2003) 'Mémoire de la Fédération des médecins spécialistes du Québec: Projet de Loi n° 25, Loi sur les agences de développement de réseaux locaux de services se danté et de services sociaux', Présenté à la Commission des affaires sociales, 2 décembre.

FMSQ (2006) 'Un financement du système de santé public fort, sans argent? La FMSQ s'étonne', 4 avril.

FMSQ (2014) 'Mémoire de la Fédération des médecins spécialistes du Québec. Projet de loi n° 10: Loi modifiant l'organisation et la gouvernance du réseau de la santé et des services sociaux notamment par l'abolition des agences régionales', CSSS – 007M CP – PL 10, Abolition des agences régionales, Déposé à la Commission de la santé et des services sociaux, 20 octobre.

FMSQ (2015a) '50 ans Fédération des médecins spécilaistes du Québec', *Le Spécialiste*, 17, numéro hors série, décembre.

FMSQ (2015b) 'Mémoire de la Fédération des médecins spécialistes du Québec, Projet de loi n° 20: Loi édictant la Loi favorisant l'accès aux services de médecine de famille et de médecine spécialisée et modifiant diverses dispositions législatives en matière de procréation assistée', CSSS – 038M, CP – PL 20, Accès services de médecine, Déposé à la Commission de la santé et des services sociaux, 17 mars.

FMSQ (2017) 'Mémoire de la Fédération des médecins spécialistes du Québec, Projet de loi n° 130: Loi modifiant certaines dispositions relatives à l'organisation clinique et à la gestion des établissements de santé et de services sociaux', CSSS – 010M, CP – PL 130, Organisation clinique, Déposé à la Commission de la santé et des services sociaux, 14 février.

Ford-Gilboe, M., Wathen, C.N., Varcoe, C., Herbert, C., Jackson, B.E., Lavoie, J.G. et al (2018) 'How equity-oriented health care affects health: Key mechanisms and implications for primary health care practice and policy', *The Milbank Quarterly*, 96(4): 635–71.

Forest, P.G. and Denis, J.L. (2012) 'Real reform in health systems: An introduction', *Journal of Health Politics, Policy and Law*, 37(4): 575–86.

Forest, P.G. and Martin, D. (2018) *Fit for Purpose: Findings and Recommendations of the External Review of the Pan-Canadian Health Organizations: Summary Report*, Ottawa, ON: Health Canada.

Fournier, M.A. (2001) 'Les politiques de main-d'oeuvre médicale au Québec: Bilan 1970–2000', *Ruptures: Revue transdisciplinaire en sante*, 7(2): 79–98.

Fournier, M.A. and Contandriopoulos, A.P. (1997) 'Les effectifs médicaux au Québec: Mieux comprendre le passé pour envisager l'avenir, situation de 1980 à 1994 et projections pour les années 2000', Groupe de recherche interdisciplinaire en santé, Université de Montréal.

Fox, T. (1950) 'Mechanism and purpose', *The Lancet*, 1: 27.

Fox, T. (1976) 'Industrial action, the national health service, and the medical profession', *The Lancet*, 23(2): 892–5.

Fredman, S. and Morris, G. (1989) *The State as Employer: Labour Law in the Public Service*, London and New York: Mansell.

Freemantle, N., Richardson, M., Wood, J., Ray, D., Khosla, S., Shahian, D. et al (2012) 'Weekend hospitalization and additional risk of death: An analysis of inpatient data', *Journal of the Royal Society of Medicine*, 105: 74–84.

Freidson, E. (1974) *Professional Dominance: The Social Structure of Medical Care*, New Jersey, NJ: Transaction Publishers.

Freidson, E. (1983) 'The reorganization of the professions by regulation', *Law and Human Behavior*, 7(2–3): 279.

Freidson, E. (1985) 'The reorganization of the medical profession', *Medical Care Review*, 42(1): 11–35.

Freidson, E. (1988) *Profession of Medicine: A Study of the Sociology of Applied Knowledge*, Chicago, IL: University of Chicago Press.

Freidson, E. (1994) *Professionalism Reborn: Theory, Prophecy, and Policy*, Chicago, IL: University of Chicago Press.

Freidson, E. (2001) *Professionalism, the Third Logic: On the Practice of Knowledge*, Chicago, IL: University of Chicago Press.

Friedman, C.P., Allee, N.J., Delaney, B.C., Flynn, A.J., Silverstein, J.C., Sullivan, K. and Young, K.A. (2017) 'The science of Learning Health Systems: Foundations for a new journal', *Learning Health Systems*, 1(1): e10020.

Garant, P. (2017) *Droit administratif* (7th edn), Montreal: Thomson Reuters.

Gemine, R., Davies G.R., Tarrant, S., Davies, R.M., James, M. and Lewis, K.E. (2021) 'Factors associated with work-related burnout in NHS staff during COVID-19: A cross-sectional mixed methods study', BMJ Open. Available at: https://bmjopen.bmj.com/content/11/1/e042591

General Medical Services Committee (1986) *Report to a Special Conference of Representatives of Local Medical Committees on 13 November 1986*, London: BMA.

General Medical Services Committee (1989) *Report to a Special Conference of Representatives of Local Medical Committees on 21/22 June 1989*, London: BMA.

General Medical Services Committee (1990) *Report to a Special Conference of Representatives of Local Media Committees on 21 March 1990*, London: BMA.

Germain, S. (2019) *Justice and Profit in Healthcare Law: A Comparative Analysis of the United States and the United Kingdom*, London: Hart Publishing.

Germain, S. (2021) 'The role of medical professionals in shaping healthcare law during COVID-19', *Amicus Curiae*, 3(1): 33–55.

Germain, S. and Yong, A. (2020) 'COVID-19 highlighting inequalities in access to healthcare in England: A case study of ethnic minority and migrant women', *Feminist Legal Studies*, 28: 301–10.

Germain, S. and Yong, S. (2021a) *Written Evidence from the Gender & Sexualities Research Centre (GSRC) at City, University of London for Women's Health Strategy*, City Law School Working Paper 2021/05.

Germain, S. and Yong, A. (2021b: forthcoming) 'Ethnic minority and migrant women's struggles in accessing healthcare during COVID-19: An intersectional analysis', *Journal of Cultural Research*.

Gerth, H.H. and Wright Mills, C. (eds) (1948) *From Max Weber: Essays in Sociology*, New York: Oxford University Press.

Gillett, J., Hutchison, B., and Birch, S. (2001) 'Capitation and primary care in Canada: Financial incentives and the evolution of health service organizations', *International Journal of Health Services*, 31(3): 583–603.

Gingras, P. (1982) 'Les médecins lancent la guerre des chiffres', *La Presse*, 17 mai.

Giroux, M., Rocher, G. and Lajoie, A. (1999) 'L'émergence de la Loi sur les services de santé et les services sociaux de 1991: Une chronologie des événements', *Revue juridique thémis*, 33(3): 659–95.

Glennerster, H. (1995) *British Social Policy since 1945*, Oxford: Blackwell.

The Globe and Mail (1966) 'OMA pamphlet urges doctors bypass OMSIP.'

Godber, G. (1975) *The Health Service: Past, Present and Future*, London: The Athlone Press.

Godlee, F. (2012) 'The NHS is heading down a hole – should we stop digging?', *British Medical Journal*, 344: e805.

Goldman, B. (1991) 'OMA agreement signals cooperation with government, disagreement among doctors', *Canadian Medical Association Journal*, 145(2): 145–6.

Goodwin, M. (2012) 'It's representational rights, duh', *Medical Post*, 48(12): 13.

Gordon, A. and Dunlop, M. (1982) 'Ontario doctors to stage one-day protest on pay', *Toronto Star*, 27 January.

Gouldner, A.W. (1957) 'Cosmopolitans and locals: Toward an analysis of latent social roles. I', *Administrative Science Quarterly*, 2(3): 281–306.

Gouldner, A.W. (1958) 'Cosmopolitans and locals: Toward an analysis of latent social roles. II', *Administrative Science Quarterly*, 2(4): 444–80.

Grabham, T. (1994) 'Divided we fall (yet again)', *British Medical Journal*, 309: 1100–1.

Grant, K. (2015) 'Ontario slashes fees it pays to doctors following negotiations', *The Globe and Mail*, 15 January.

Greener, I. (2002) 'Understanding NHS reform: The policy-transfer, social learning, and path-dependency perspectives', *Governance*, 15: 161–83.

Greener, I. (2005) 'The role of the patient in healthcare reform: Customer, consumer or creator?', in S. Dawson and C. Sausmann (eds) *Future Health Organisations and Systems*, Basingstoke: Palgrave, pp 227–45.

Greener, I. (2006) 'Where are the medical voices raised in protest?', *BMJ*, 333: 660.

Greener, I. (2009) *Public Management: A Critical Text*, London: Palgrave Macmillan.

Greener, I. and Harrington, B.E. (2014) *Reforming Healthcare: What's the Evidence?*, Bristol: Policy Press.

Greenwood, R. and Suddaby, R. (2006) 'Institutional entrepreneurship in mature fields: The big five accounting firms', *Academy of Management Journal*, 49(1): 27–48.

Greenwood, R., Oliver, C., Sahin, K. and Suddaby, R. (2008) 'Introduction', in R. Greenwood, C. Oliver, K. Sahlin and R. Suddaby (eds) *The SAGE Handbook of Organizational Institutionalism*, London, Thousand Oaks, New Dehli, Singapore: SAGE Publications Ltd, pp 1–46.

Greenwood, R., Raynard, M., Kodeih, F., Micelotta, E.R. and Lounsbury, M. (2011) 'Institutional complexity and organizational responses', *Academy of Management Annals*, 5(1): 317–71.

Greer, H. (1966) 'Ontario medicare now law', *Toronto Star*, 18 February.

Greer, H. (1966) 'Ontario yields on Medicare, accepts compulsory coverage', *Toronto Star*, 26 October.

Gruen, R.L., Campbell, E.G. and Blumenthal, D. (2006) 'Public roles of US physicians: Community participation, political involvement, and collective advocacy', *Journal of the American Medical Association*, 296(20): 2467–75.

Guardian, The (2015) 'Junior doctors to be balloted for strike action, says British Medical Association', 26 September.

Guindon, H. (1998) 'Chronique de l'évolution sociale et politique du Québec depuis 1945', *Cahiers de recherche sociologique*, 30: 33–78.

Gunz, H.P. and Gunz, S.P. (2006) 'Professional ethics in formal organizations', in *Professional Service Firms* (pp 257–81), Bingley: Emerald Group Publishing Limited.

Hafferty, F.W. and Light, D.W. (1995) 'Professional dynamics and the changing nature of medical work', *Journal of Health and Social Behavior*, 'Extra Issue: Forty Years of Medical Sociology: The State of the Art and Directions for the Future': 132–53.

Hafferty, F.W. and Castellani, B. (2011) 'Two cultures: Two ships: The rise of a professionalism movement within modern medicine and medical sociology's disappearance from the professionalism debate', in B.A. Pescosolido, J.K. Martin, J.D. McLeod and J.D. Rogers (eds) *Handbook of the Sociology of Health, Illness, and Healing*, New York: Springer, pp 201–19.

Halcrow, M. (1989) *Keith Joseph: A Single Mind*, London: Macmillan.

Haliechuk, R. (1981) 'Ontario told to ban MD's extra billing or face cash loss', *Toronto Star*, 18 October.

Hallett vs Derby Hospitals NHS Foundation Trust, Neutral Citation Number [2018] EWHC 796 (QB) (2018).

Ham, C. (2000) *The Politics of NHS Reforms 1988-1997*, London: The King's Fund.

Ham, C. (2009) *Health Policy in Britain*, London: Palgrave Macmillan.

Ham, C., Clark, J. and Spurgeon, J. (2011) *Medical Leadership: From Dark Side to Centre Stage*, London: The King's Fund.

Harrington, D. (1985a) 'Liberals, NDP sign a pact, but Peterson says I'm the boss', *Toronto Star*, 29 May.

Harrington, D. (1985b) 'Ready to deliver the prescription', *Toronto Star*, 20 July.

Harrington, D. (1986) 'Negotiate an end to extra-billing Elston urges doctors', *Toronto Star*, 4 March.

Harrison, B. and Guo M. (2015) '2015 Ontario health cut backs: Overview and specific impact on primary care', *University of Ottawa Journal of Medicine*, 5(1): 21–5.

Harrison, R.G. (1993) 'Hybrids and hybrid zones: Historical perspective', in R.G. Harrison (ed) *Hybrid Zones and the Evolutionary Process*, Oxford: Oxford University Press, pp 3–12.

Harrison, S. and Pollitt, C. (1994) *Controlling Health Professionals*, Buckingham: Open University Press.

Haug, M.R. (1972) 'Deprofessionalization: An alternate hypothesis for the future', *The Sociological Review*, 20(S1): 195–211.

Haug, M.R. (1988) 'A re-examination of the hypothesis of physician deprofessionalization', *The Milbank Quarterly*, 66(S2): 48–56.

Health and Social Care Act (2012) *Health and Social Care Act*, London: HMSO.

Health Foundation (2020) *Building Back Fairer: The Covid-19 Marmot Review*, London: Health Foundation.

Hebdon, B. and Warrian, P. (1999) 'Coercive bargaining: Public sector restructuring under the Ontario Social Contract, 1993–1996', *ILR Review*, 52(2): 196–212.

Heller, L. (1979) 'Exodus – and doctors blame status not greed', *Toronto Star*, 14 March.

Henderich, J. (1979) 'Bégin blames "stingy" fees for doctors quitting OHIP', *Toronto Star*, 14 March.

Hinings, C.R. (2005) 'The professions', in S. Ackroyd, P. Batt, P. Thompson and P.S. Tolbert (eds) *The Oxford Handbook of Work and Organisation*, Oxford: Oxford University Press, pp 485–507.

Hinsliff-Smith, K., Gordon, A., Devi, R. and Goodman, C. (2020) 'The COVID-19 pandemic in UK care homes: Revealing the cracks in the system', *The Journal of Nursing Home Research Science*, 2020(6): 58–60.

HM Government (2010) *The Coalition: Our Programme for Government*, London: Cabinet Office.

Hodges, D. (2005) 'Web tool gauges efficiency of Ont. cancer care', *Medical Post*, 41(18): 10 May.

Hollobon, J. (1968) 'Leave public attitudes to public, Ontario Medical Association told', *The Globe and Mail*.

Holloran, S.T. (1990) 'The federal government, Ontario and medical care insurance: A study in federal provincial relations', Electronic Theses and Dissertations, 3996.

Honigsbaum, F. (1989) *Health, Happiness and Security: The Creation of the National Health Service*, Abingdon: Routlege.

Hood, C. (1983) *The Tools of Government*, London: Macmillan.

House of Commons (1946) Second Reading of the NHS Bill.

House of Commons (1989a) Second Reading of the White Paper *Working for Patients*.

House of Commons (1989b) Second Reading of the NHS Community and Care Bill.

House of Commons (2010) Health Committee.

House of Lords (1973) Second Reading of the NHS Reorganisation Bill.

House of Lords (2007) *Companion to the Standing Orders and Proceedings of the House of Lords*, Appendix E.

House of Lords (2011) Second Reading of the Health and Social Care Bill.

Howlett, M. (2012) 'The lessons of failure: learning and blame avoidance in public policy-making', *International Political Science Review*, 33(5): 539–55.

Howlett, M., Kekez, A. and Poocharoen, O.O. (2017) 'Understanding co-production as a policy tool: Integrating new public governance and comparative policy theory', *Journal of Comparative Policy Analysis: Research and Practice*, 19(5): 487–501.

Hunter, D.J. (2016) *The Health Debate*, Bristol: Policy Press.

Hwang, H. and Powell, W.W. (2005) 'Institutions and entrepreneurship', in S.A. Alvarez, R. Agarwal and O. Sorenson (eds) *Handbook of Entrepreneurship Research*, Cham: Springer, pp 201–32.

Iacobucci, G. (2014) 'NHS England's five year plan', *British Medical Journal*, 349: g6484.

Iacobucci, G. (2015) 'Tackle shortfall in NHS funding, healthcare leaders tell health secretary', *British Medical Journal*, 350: h2577.

Immergut, E.M. (1990) 'Institutions, veto points, and policy results: A comparative analysis of health care', *Journal of Public Policy*, 10(4): 391–416.

Irvine, D. (1999) 'The performance of doctors: The new professionalism', *The Lancet*, 353: 1174–7.

Jensen, L.S. (2008) 'Government, the State, and governance polity', *Polity*, 40(3): 379–85.

Jessop, B. (2011) 'The state: Government and governance', in A. Pike, A. Rodríguez-Pose and J. Tomaney (eds) *Handbook of Local and Regional Development* (2nd edn), London: Routledge, pp 239–41.

Johns, G. (2006) 'The essential impact of context on organizational behavior', *Academy of Management Review*, 31(2): 386–408.

Johnson, T. (1972) 'Imperialism and the professions: Notes on the development of professional occupations in Britain's colonies and the New States', *The Sociological Review*, 20(1_suppl): 281–309.

Johnson, T., Larkin, G. and Saks, M. (1995) 'Governmentality and the institutionalization of expertise', in T. Johnson, G. Larkin and M. Saks (eds) *Health Professions and the State in Europe*, Abingdon: Routledge, pp 11–20.

Jones, C. (1950) *Enquiry into the Financial Working of the Service*, CAB 134/518, PRO.

Jones, H. (2014) *Health and Society in Twentieth Century Britain*, Abingdon: Routledge.

Judge, K. and Solomon, M. (1993) 'Public opinion and the National Health Service: Patterns and perspectives in consumer satisfaction', *Journal of Social Policy*, 22: 299–327.

Justice for Health Ltd, R (On the Application Of) vs The Secretary of State for Health (2016).

Kahn-Freund, O. (1972) *Labour and the Law*, London: Stevens & Sons Ltd.

Kaissi, A. (2014) 'Enhancing physician engagement: An international perspective', *International Journal of Health Services*, 44(3): 567–92.

Kavanagh, D. and Morris, P. (1989) *Consensus Politics from Attlee to Thatcher*, Oxford: Blackwell.

Kennedy, I. (2001) *Learning from Bristol: The Report of the Public Inquiry into Children's Heart Surgery at the Bristol Royal Infirmary, 1984–95*, London: The Stationery Office.

The King's Fund (2015) *The NHS under the Coalition Government Part One: NHS Reform*, London: The King's Fund.

Kitchener, M., Caronna, C.A. and Shortell, S.M. (2005) 'From the doctor's workshop to the iron cage? Evolving modes of physician control in US health systems', *Social Science & Medicine*, 60(6): 1311–22.

Klein, R. (1990) 'The state and the profession: The politics of the double bed', *BMJ*, 301: 700–2.

Klein, R. (2013) *The New Politics of the NHS: From Creation to Reinvention* (7th edn), Abingdon: Routledge.

Klein, R. (2018) 'The National Health Service (NHS) at 70: Bevan's double-edged legacy', *Health Economics, Policy and Law*, 14(1): 1–10.

Kleinert, S. and Horton, R. (2017) 'From universal health coverage to right care for health', *The Lancet*, 390(10090): 101–2.

Kmietowicz, Z. (2003) 'Consultants threaten strike over contract stalemate', *British Medical Journal*, 326: 1165.

Kmietowicz, Z. (2005) 'GMC gives evidence to inquiry', *British Medical Journal*, 330: 1044.

Kondro, W. (2007) 'Ontario overhauls medical audit regime', *Canadian Medical Association Journal*, 177(4): 334.

Koul, S. (2012) 'Shoot-out at the OMA corral', *Medical Post*, 48(9): 10.

Kralj, B. and Barber, J. (2013) 'Physician payment reform – part II: Implementation of episode bundling/quality based procedures', *Ontario Medical Review*, 21–5.

La Presse (1970) 'Les omnipraticiens signent leur convention collective', 12 novembre, A1, A6.

La Presse (2002) 'Un décès ne fait pas reculer l'hôpital de Shawinigan. Les urgences fermés la nuit', 22 juin, A3.

La Presse (2015a) Publicity by FMOQ, 24 February, A6

La Presse (2015b) Publicity by FMOQ, 27 February, A5.

La Presse (2015c) Publicity by FMOQ, 21 March, A6.

Lacoursier, A. (2015) 'Projet de loi 20: La grogne s'installe chez les médecins', *La Presse*, 26 mars.

The Lancet (1971) 'Invitation to counsult', 297: 1056.

Langley, A. (1999) 'Strategies for theorizing from process data', *Academy of Management Review*, 24(4): 691–710.

Langley, A., Smallman, C., Tsoukas, H. and van de Ven, A.H. (2013) 'Process studies of change in organization and management: Unveiling temporality, activity, and flow', *Academy of Management Journal*, 56(1): 1–13.

Lansley, A. (2005) 'The future of health and public service regulation', Speech, NHS Confederation.

Larson, L.M. (1977) *The Rise of Professionalism: A Sociological Analysis*, Berkeley, CA: University of California.

Larson, M.S. (1979) 'Professionalism: Rise and fall', *International Journal of Health Services*, 9(4): 607–27.

Lascoumes, P. and Le Galès, P. (2004) *Gouverner par les instruments*, Paris: Presses de Sciences po.

Lascoumes, P. and Le Galès, P. (2007) 'Introduction: Understanding public policy through its instruments – from the nature of instruments to the sociology of public policy instrumentation', *Governance*, 20(1): 1–21.

Lascoumes, P. and Le Galès, P. (2010) 'Instrument', in L. Boussaguet, S. Jacquot and P. Ravinet (eds) *Dictionnaire des politiques publiques* (vol 3), Paris: Presses de Sciences Po, pp 325–35.

Laugesen, M.J. (2016) *Fixing Medical Prices*, Cambridge, MA: Harvard University Press.

Lazar, H., Forest, P. G., Church, J. and Lavis, J. N. (eds) (2013) *Paradigm Freeze: Why It Is So Hard to Reform Health Care in Canada*, Montréal, QC: McGill-Queen's Press.

Le Devoir (2002) 'Legault sonne la fin de la récréation: Le ministre de la santé est prêt à se heurter aux médecins pour "préserver le système"', 25 juillet.

Lee-Potter, J. (1997) *A Damn Bad Business: The NHS Deformed*, London: Gollancz.

Leicht, K.T. (2005) 'Professions', in G. Ritzer (ed) *Encyclopedia of Social Theory*, London: SAGE Publications Ltd, pp 603–6.

Leicht, K.T. and Fennell, M.L. (1997) 'The changing organizational context of professional work', *Annual Review of Sociology*, 23(1): 215–31.

Leicht, K.T. and Fennell, M.L. (2008) 'Institutionalism and the professions', in R. Greenwood, C. Oliver, R. Suddaby and K. Sahlin Anderson (eds) *Handbook of Organizational Institutionalism*, Thousand Oaks, CA: SAGE Publications Ltd, pp 431–48.

Lemke, T. (2007) 'An indigestible meal? Foucault, governmentality and state theory', *Distinktion: Scandinavian Journal of Social Theory*, 8(2), 43–64.

Leslie, C. (2013a) 'Behind the scenes of OMA fee talks', *Medical Post*, 49(16): 14.

Leslie, C. (2013b) 'The income-raising role of medical associations', *Medical Post*, 49(18): 14.

Leslie, C. (2015a) '2 negotiations. The timeline, the players', *Medical Post*, 51(2): 22.

Leslie, C. (2015b) 'It's time to get back to the negotiating table in Ontario', *Medical Post*, 51(6): 6.

Leslie, C. (2016) 'The road to binding arbitration', *Medical Post*, 52(4): 4.

Lewis, S. (2015) 'A system in name only: Access, variation, and reform in Canada's provinces', *New England Journal of Medicine*, 372(6): 497–500.

Light, D. (1995) 'Countervailing powers', in T. Johnson, G. Larkin and M. Saks (eds) *Health Professions and the State in Europe*, London: Routledge, pp 25–41.

Linder, S.H. and Peters, B.G. (1989) 'Instruments of government: Perceptions and contexts', *Journal of Public Policy*, 9: 35–58.

Littler, C.R. (1990) 'The labour process debate: A theoretical teview 1974–88', in D. Knights and H. Willmott (eds) *Labour Process Theory*, London: Palgrave Macmillan, pp 46–94.

Lodge, M. (2008) 'Regulation, the regulatory state and European politics', *West European Politics*, 31(1–2): 280–301.

Loudon, I., Horder, J. and Webster, C. (1998) *General Practice under the National Health Service, 1948–1997*, Oxford: Clarendon Press.

Lowe, R. (1998) *The Welfare State in Britain since 1945*, Basingstoke: Macmillan International Higher Education.

Macdonald, K.M. (1995) *The Sociology of the Professions*, London: SAGE Publications.

Mackenzie, H. (2010) *Steering Ontario Out of Recession: A Plan of Action*, Technical Paper: Ontario Budget 2010, Canadian Centre for Policy Alternatives.

Maioni, A. (1997) 'Parting at the crossroads: The development of health insurance in Canada and the United States, 1940–1965', *Comparative Politics*, 411–31.

Maioni, A. (2004) 'New century, new risks: The Marsh Report and the post-war welfare state in Canada', *Policy Options – Montreal*, 25(7): 20.

Malling, E. (1970) 'Special report: 60% of Ontario doctors accept medicare rates', *Toronto Star*, 10 October.

Manthorpe, J. (1979) 'Ontario puts the boot to physicians' union – but gently, gently', *Toronto Star*, 31 March.

Marchildon, G.P. (2013) 'Canada: Health system review', *Health System in Transition*, 15(1): 1–179.

Marchildon, G.P. and Hutchison, B. (2016) 'Primary care in Ontario, Canada: New proposals after 15 years of reform', *Health Policy*, 120(7): 732–8.

Marcus, L.J., Dorn, B.C. and McNulty, E.J. (2011) *Renegotiating Health Care: Resolving Conflict to Build Collaboration* (2nd edn), San Francisco, CA: Jossey-Bass Publishers.

Marin S. (2017) 'Les Médecins spécialistes exigent le retrait du projet de loi 130', *Le Soleil*, 25 mai.

Marmor, T. and Wendt, C. (2012) 'Conceptual frameworks for comparing healthcare politics and policy', *Health Policy*, 107(1): 11–20.

Marshall, T.H. (1939) 'The recent history of professionalism in relation to social structure and social policy', *Canadian Journal of Economics and Political Science / Revue canadienne de economiques et science politique*, 5(3): 325–40.

Martin, G.P. and Waring, J. (2018) 'Realising governmentality: Pastoral power, governmental discourse and the (re) constitution of subjectivities', *The Sociological Review*, 0038026118755616.

Martin, J.L. and Lembo, A. (2020) 'On the other side of values', *American Journal of Sociology*, 126(1): 52–98.

Mauss, M. and Durkheim, É. (1937) 'Morale professionnelle: Trois leçons extraites d'un cours d'Émile Durkheim, de morale civique et professionnelle (1898–1900)', *Revue de métaphysique et de morale*, 44(3): 527–44.

Maynard, A. (2013) 'Health care rationing: Doing it better in public and private health care systems', *Journal of Health Politics, Policy and Law*, 38(6): 1103–27.

McGivern, G., Currie, G., Ferlie, E., Fitzgerald, L. and Waring, J. (2015) 'Hybrid manager-professionals' identity work: The maintenance and hybridization of medical professionalism in managerial contexts', *Public Administration*, 93(2): 412–32.

McIver, S. (2000) 'Public consultation. Consulting room', *The Health Service Journal*, 110: 28–9.

McKinlay, J.B. and Arches, J. (1985) 'Towards the proletarianization of physicians', *International Journal of Health Services*, 15(2): 161–95.

McKinlay, J.B. and Marceau, L.D. (2002) 'The end of the golden age of doctoring', *International Journal of Health Services*, 32(2): 379–416.

McNulty, T. and Ferlie, E. (2002) *Re-engineering Health Care: The Complexities of Organizational Transformation*, Oxford: Oxford University Press.

Mechanic, D. and Rochefort, D.A. (1996) 'Comparative medical systems', *Annual Review of Sociology*, 22(1): 239–70.

Medical Post (1996a) 'Ontario doctors warming to capitation: Rostering', 32(1): 52.

Medical Post (1996b) 'OMA plots media strategy', 32(1): 6

Medical Post (1996c) 'Ontario doctors lose out in government power grab', 32(5): 1–81.

Medical Post (1996d) 'Ontario health minister Jim Wilson takes aim at misconceptions about controversial Bill 26', 32(2): 22–3.

Medical Post (1996e) 'Bill 26 will give Ontario doctors less say', 32(11): 44.

Medical Post (1997) 'Ontario's FP coalition picking up steam', 33(28): 4.

Medical Services Review Committee (1962) *A Review of the Medical Services in Great Britain: The Report of [the Medical Services Review] Committee* (Sir Arthur Porritt), Social Assay.

Meyer, J.W. (2010) 'World society, institutional theories, and the actor', *Annual Review of Sociology*, 36: 1–20.

Millin, L. (1968) 'OMA leader says Canada is communist', *The Globe and Mail*.

Milnes, A. and Zade, R. (2017) 'Acknowledgements', in D. Peterson and S. Paikin (authors) and A. Milnes and R. Zade (eds) *Without Walls or Barriers: The Speeches of Premier David Peterson*, Montréal, Kingston, London and Ithaca, NY: McGill-Queen's University Press, pp xiii–xiv.

Minister of Health (1962) *A Hospital Plan for England and Wales*, Cmnd. 1604, London: HMSO.

Ministry of Health and Department of Health for Scotland (1944) *A National Health Service: The White Paper Proposals in Brief*, London: HMSO. Available at: https://www.sochealth.co.uk/national-health-service/the-sma-and-the-foundation-of-the-national-health-service-dr-leslie-hilliard-1980/a-national-health-service/

Mintzberg, H. (1979) *The Structuring of Organizations*, Englewood Cliffs, NJ: Prentice Hall.

Mintzberg, H. and Waters, J.A. (1982) 'Tracking strategy in an entrepreneurial firm', *Academy of Management Journal*, 25: 465–99.

Mitchell, R.K., Agle, B.R. and Wood, D.J. (1997) 'Toward a theory of stakeholder identification and salience: Defining the principle of who and what really counts', *Academy of Management Review*, 22(4): 853–86.

MOHLTC (Ministry of Health and Long-Term Care) (2012) *Ontario's Action Plan for Health Care: Better Patient Care through Better Value from our Health Care Dollars*, January, Toronto: Government of Ontario.

Montagna, P.D. (1968) 'Professionalization and bureaucratization in large professional organizations', *American Journal of Sociology*, 74(2): 138–45.

Moran, M. (1995) 'Explaining change in the National Health Service: Corporatism, closure and democratic capitalism', *Public Policy and Administration*, 10: 21–33.

Morrell, D. (1998) 'Introduction and overview', in I. Loudon, J. Horder and C. Webster (eds) *General Practice under the National Heath Service 1948–1997*, London: Clarendon Press, pp 1–19.

Morrell, K. (2006) 'Policy as narrative: New Labour's reform of the National Health Service', *Public Administration*, 84(2): 367–85.

Morris, T., Greenwood, R. and Fairclough, S. (2010) 'Decision making in professional service firms', in P.C. Nutt and D.C. Wilson (eds) *Handbook of Decision Making*, New York: John Wiley & Sons, pp 276–306.

Mumby, D.K., Thomas, R., Martí, I. and Seidl, D. (2017) 'Resistance redux', *Organization Studies*, 38(9): 1157–83.

MSSS (Ministère de la Santé et des Services sociaux) (1989) 'Pour améliorer la santé et le bien-être au Québec: Orientations', Gouvernement du Québec, Ministère de la Santé et des Services sociaux avril.

MSSS (1990) 'Une réforme axée sur le citoyen' ['A citizen-centred reform'], Gouvernement du Québec, Ministère de la Santé et des Services sociaux, décembre.

MSSS (2006) 'Garantir l'accès: un défi d'équité , d'efficience et de qualité', Gouvernement du Québec, Ministère de la Santé et des Services sociaux fevrier.

Muncin, C. (1997) 'Sinclair sets sights on primary-care reform', *Medical Post*, 33(34): 4.

Muzio, D. and Kirkpatrick, I. (2011) 'Introduction: Professions and organizations – A conceptual framework', *Current Sociology*, 59(4): 389–405.

Muzio, D., Brock, D.M. and Suddaby, R. (2013) 'Professions and institutional change: Towards an institutionalist sociology of the professions', *Journal of Management Studies*, 50(5): 699–721.

Nadeau, J. (2015a) 'Le Barreau et la FMOQ refusent de comparaître tant qu'ils ne seront pas prêts', *Le Devoir*, 24 février.

Nadeau, J. (2015b) 'Duel épique pour une réforme condamnée', *Le Devoir*, 18 mars.

Nadeau, J. (2015c) 'Les omnipraticiens veulent négocier en privé', *Le Devoir*, 19 mars.

NAHA (National Association of Health Authorities for England and Wales) (1987) *Autumn Survey*.

Nairne, P. (1983) 'Managing the DHSS elephant: Reflections on a giant department Sir Patrick Nairne', *The Political Quarterly*, 54: 243–56.

NAO (National Audit Office) (2007) *Pay Modernisation: A New Contract for NHS Consultants in England*, London: NAO.

National Assembly Debates (1970a) Assemblée nationale, Journal des débats, Commission permanente de la santé, 7 juillet, 10(21). Available at: http://www.assnat.qc.ca/fr/travaux-parlementaires/commissions/cs-4-avant-1984-29-1/journal-debats/CS-700707.html?appelant=MC.

National Assembly Debates (1970b) Assemblée nationale, Journal des débats, Commission permanente de la santé, 1 octobre, 10(29); Fascicule n°22, 15 octobre, pp 1385–436.

National Assembly Debates (1990) Assemblée nationale, Journal des débats, Commission permanente des affaires sociales, 19 mars, 31(64): 8, 9.

National Assembly Debates (2015a) Bill 20, 17 mars, 44(40).

National Assembly Debates (2015b) 19 mars, 44(42).

National Housing Federation (2020) *Housing, Communities and Local Government Committee Inquiry into the Impact of COVID-19 (Coronavirus) on Homelessness and the Private Rented Sector*, London, National Housing Federation Limited.

Nettl, J.P. (1968) 'The State as a conceptual variable', *World Politics*, 20: 559–63.

Newbery, L. (1980) 'Doctors' check-up gets college okay', *Toronto Star*, 3 July.

Newbery, L. (1986) 'Here are the issues', *Toronto Star*, 15 June.

NHS England (2014) 'Five year forward view', NHS England.

NHS Future Forum (2011) *Summary Report on Proposed Changes to the NHS*.

Noel, A. (1987) 'Les résidents et internes rentrent au travail', *La Presse*, 18 novembre.

Noordegraaf, M. (2011) 'Risky business: How professionals and professional fields (must) deal with organizational issues', *Organization Studies*, 32(10): 1349–71.

Noordegraaf, M. (2013) 'Reconfiguring professional work: Changing forms of professionalism in public services', *Administration & Society*, 48(7): 783–810.

Noordegraaf, M. (2015) 'Hybrid professionalism and beyond: (New) Forms of public professionalism in changing organizational and societal contexts', *Journal of Professions and Organization*, 2(2): 187–206.

O'Donnell, J. (1979) 'I'm not a money-grubber', *Toronto Star*, 6 January.

OMA (Ontario Medical Association) (2009) Submission to the Standing Committee on Social Policy on Bill 179: 'An Act to Amend Regulated Health Professions Statutes', 16 September.

OMSIP (1967) 'OMSIP progress report: Most MDs back plan, Dymond says', *The Globe and Mail*. Available at: https://search.proquest.com/hnpg lobeandmail/docview/1270026443/abstract/120703C2716142BEPQ/5

Oppenheimer, M. (1972) 'The proletarianization of the professional', *The Sociological Review*, 20(1_suppl): 213–27.

Ouellet, M. (2014) 'Réforme en santé: un projet de loi irrecevable, selon les médecins spécialistes', *Le Devoir*, 20 octobre.

Pal, L. (2006) *Beyond Policy Analysis – Public Issue Management in Turbulent Times*, Toronto: Nelson Education.

Paradeise, C. (1988) 'Les professions comme marchés du travail fermés', *Sociologie et sociétés*, 20(2): 9–21.

Paré, I. (1991) 'Un placard qui choque', *Le Devoir*, 8 juin.

Paré, I. (1996) 'Le branle-bas de combat à l'hôpital Notre-Dame: Les médecins rejettent toute nouvelle compression', *Le Devoir*, 15 juin.

Parkin, F. (1979) *The Marxist Theory of Class: A Bourgeois Critique*, London: Tavistock.

Parliament (1948) *Report of the Inter-Departmental Committee on Remuneration of General Practitioners*, Cmd 6810, London: HMSO.

Parsons, T. (1939) 'The professions and social structure', *Social Forces*, 17(4): 457–67.

Parsons, T. (1954) 'Professional and social structure', in T. Parsons (ed) *Essays in Sociological Theory*, Glencoe, IL: Free Press, pp 34–49.

Patel, K. and Rushefsky, M.E. (2014) *Healthcare Politics and Policy in America* (4th edn), Armonk, NY: ME Sharpe.

Pater, J.E. (1981) *The Making of the National Service*, London: Pitman's Medical.

Pettigrew, A.M. (1987) 'Context and action in the transformation of the firm', *Journal of Management Studies*, 24: 649–70.

Pettigrew, A.M. (1992) 'The character and significance of strategy process research', *Strategic Management Journal*, 13(S2): 5–16.

Pettigrew, A.M. (2012) 'Context and action in the transformation of the firm: A reprise', *Journal of Management Studies*, 49(7): 1304–28.

Pettigrew, A.M., Woodman, R.W. and Cameron, K.S. (2001) 'Studying organizational change and development: Challenges for future research', *Academy of Management Journal*, 44(4): 697–713.

Pierson, P. (2011) 'The welfare state over the very long run', *ZeS-Arbeitspapier*, No. 02/2011, Bremen: Universität Bremen, Zentrum für Sozialpolitik (ZeS).

Pildes, R.H. and Sunstein, C.R. (1995) 'Reinventing the regulatory state', *The University of Chicago Law Review*, 62(1): 1–129.

Platt, S. (1998) 'Government by task force', *Catalyst Paper*, 2.

Pole, K. (2004) 'Money gets cautious nod from health groups', *Medical Post*, 40(36): 1.

Pollitt, C. (1993) *Managerialism and the Public Services: Cuts or Cultural Change in the 1990s?*, Oxford: Blackwell Business.

Pollitt, C. and Bouckaert, G. (2017) *Public Management Reform: A Comparative Analysis – Into the Age of Austerity*, Oxford: Oxford University Press.

Pollock, A.M., Price, D., Viebrock, E., Miller, E. and Watt, G. (2007) 'The market in primary care', *British Medical Journal*, 335: 475–7.

Pomey, M.P., Denis, J.L. and Dumez, V. (eds) (2019) *Patient Engagement: How Patient–Provider Partnerships Transform Healthcare Organizations*, Springer Nature.

Porter, M.E. (2009) 'A strategy for health care reform – Toward a value-based system', *The New England Journal of Medicine*, 361(2): 109–12.

Powell, M. (1998) 'In what sense a national health service?', *Public Policy and Administration*, 13: 56–69.

Power, M. (2011) 'Foucault and sociology', *Annual Review of Sociology*, 37: 35–56.

Priest, L. (1992) 'Doctors to get 1% hike under tentative agreement', *Toronto Star*, 7 October.

Priest, L. (1993a) 'New doctors fear for jobs as NDP plans to cut fees', *Toronto Star*, 1 May.

Priest, L. (1993b) 'New MDs feel betrayed as NDP plan slashes jobs', *Toronto Star*, 10 May.

Priest, L. (1993c) 'The OMA contract pill wasn't all bitter', *Toronto Star*, August 19.

Priest, L. (1993d) 'Doctors, province battle over health-care cuts', *Toronto Star*, 29 December.

Priest, L. (1994a) 'Hold off on tests, MDs tell public', *Toronto Star*, 30 November.

Priest, L. (1994b) 'Doctors lose pay', *Toronto Star*, 17 December.

Priest, L. (1996) 'Sign a deal with the doc is new health thought', *Toronto Star*, 15 February.

Public Records Office (1948) CAB 129/131.

Public Records Office (1950a) CAB 129/38.

Public Records Office (1950b) CAB 128/17.

Quadagno, J. (2005) *One Nation, Uninsured: Why the US Has No National Health Insurance*, Oxford: Oxford University Press.

Quadagno, J. (2010) 'Institutions, interest groups, and ideology: An agenda for the sociology of health care reform', *Journal of Health and Social Behavior*, 51(2): 125–36.

Rachlis, M. (2009) 'Can this minister fix the health line?', *Toronto Star*, 16 October.

Raelin, J.A. (1986) *The Clash of Cultures: Managers and Professionals*, Cambridge, MA: Harvard Business Press.

Raine, K., Hernandez, C., Nykiforuk, C., Reed, S., Montemurro, G., Lytvyak, E. and MacLellan-Wright, M.-F. (2014) 'Measuring the process of capacity building in the Alberta Policy Coalition for Cancer Prevention', *Health Promotion Practice*, 15(4): 496–505.

Raz, J. (1986) *The Morality of Freedom*, Oxford: Clarendon Press.

Reed, M.I. (1996) 'Expert power and control in late modernity: An empirical review and theoretical synthesis', *Organization Studies*, 17(4): 573–97.

Reed, R.R. and Evans, D. (1987) 'The deprofessionalization of medicine', *Journal of the American Medical Association*, 258(22): 3279–82.

Régis, C. (2008) 'Valeur de l'imputabilité dans l'allocation des ressources au Canada: Une perspective de politiques publiques', *McGill Journal of Law & Health*, 2: 47.

Renaud, M. (1981) 'Les réformes québécoises de la santé ou les aventures d'un État narcissique', in L. Bozzini, M. Renaud, D. Gaucher and J. Llambias-Wolff (eds) *Médecine et société. Les années 80*, Montréal, QC: Les Éditions coopératives Albert Saint-Martin, pp 513–49.

Rhodes, R.A.W. (1996) 'The new governance: Governing without government', *Political Studies*, 44(4): 652–67.

Richard, P. (1971) 'Les médecins réclament des pouvoirs de contrôle', *Le Devoir*, 16 septembre.

Richardson, K. (1997) 'Go-slow approach urged on primary care reform', *Medical Post*, 33(27): 61.

Richer, J. (2016) 'Barrette serre un peu plus la vis aux médecins', *Le Devoir*, 10 décembre.

Rintala, M. (2003) *Creating the National Health Service: Aneurin Bevan and the Medical Lords*, London: Frank Cass.

Rivett, G. (1998) *From Cradle to Grave: Fifty Years of the NHS*, London: The King's Fund.

Roberge, H. (1982a) 'Les résidents et internes accusent Québec de leur 'tirer dans le dos', *La Presse*, 27 mai.

Roberge, H. (1982b) 'Entente avec les spécialistes. La loi accorde $91,647 aux omnipraticiens', *La Presse*, 22 juin.

Robertson, D. (2002) *A Dictionary of Modern Politics* (3rd edn), London and New York: Europa Publications.

Robinson, R. (1988) *Health Finance: Assessing the Options*, London: The King's Fund.

Roche, W. (2018) 'Medical regulation for the public interest in United Kingdom', in J.M. Chamberlain, M. Dent and M. Saks (eds) *Professional Health Regulation in the Public Interest: International Perspectives*, Bristol: Policy Press, pp 77–92.

Rocher, G. (2008) 'Les réformes: Une perspective sociologique', in P. Laborier, P. Noreau, M. Rioux and G. Rocher (eds) *Les réformes en santé et en justice: Le droit et la gouvernance*, Québec: Les Presses de l'Université Laval, pp 9–22.

Romanow, R.J. (2002) *Building on Values: The Future of Health Care in Canada* (Romanow Report), The Romanow Commission, Saskatoon, Saskatchewan: Privy Council

Rose, N. and Miller, P. (2010) 'Political power beyond the State: Problematics of government', *The British Journal of Sociology*, 61: 271–303.

Rose, N., O'Malley, P. and Valverde, M. (2006) 'Governmentality', *Annual Review of Law and Social Science*, 2: 83–104.

Roy, M. (1970) 'Front commun des grandes centrales syndicales contre le projet loi de l'assurance-maladie', *Le Devoir*, 30 juin.

RCP (Royal College of Physicians) (2013) *Future Hospital Commission*, London: RCP.

RCP (2017) *NHS Reality Check: Delivering Care under Pressure*, London: RCP.

RCP (2020) 'Ethical guidance published for frontline staff dealing with pandemic.' Available at: www.rcplondon.ac.uk/news/ ethical-guidance-published-frontline-staff-dealing-pandemic

Royal Commission on Doctors' and Dentists' Remuneration (1960) 'The report of the Royal Commission on Doctors' and Dentists' Remuneration', *The Journal of the College of General Practitioners*, 3: 133–4.

Royal Commission on the National Health Service (1979) *Royal Commission on the National Health Service (Merrison Commission): Record*, Cmnd 7615, London: HMSO.

Ryan, C. (1970) 'Les centrales syndicales et le projet Castonguay', *Le Devoir*, 2 juillet.

Saks, M. (1995) *Professions and the Public Interest: Medical Power, Altruism and Alternative Medicine*, Abingdon: Routledge.

Saks, M. (2010) 'Analyzing the professions: The case for the neo-Weberian approach', *Comparative Sociology*, 9(6): 887–915.

Saks, M. (2012) 'Defining a profession: The role of knowledge and expertise', *Professions and Professionalism*, 2(1): 1–10.

Saks, M. (2016) 'Professions and power: A review of theories of professions and power', in M. Dent, L. Bourgeault, J.-L. Denis and E. Kuhlmann (eds) *The Routledge Companion to the Professions and Professionalism*, Abingdon: Routledge, pp 89–104.

Saks, M. and Adams, T.L. (2019) 'Neo-Weberianism, professional formation and the state: Inside the black box', *Professions and Professionalism*, 9(2): 3190.

Salamon, L.M. (ed) (2002) *The Tools of Government: A Guide to the New Governance*, New York: Oxford University Press.

Salter, B. (2004) *The New Politics of Medicine*, Basingstoke: Palgrave Macmillan.

Saltman, R.B. (2018) 'Foreword', in J.M. Chamberlain, M. Dent and M. Saks (eds) *Professional Health Regulation in the Public Interest: International Perspectives*, Bristol: Policy Press, pp xi–xiii.

Samuels, A. (2018) 'A constitutional statute?', *Statute Law Review*, 1.

Savard, A.-M. (2017) 'Les médecins comme travailleurs autonomes au sein du système public de santé au Québec: Le passage d'une autonomie professionnelle à une imputabilité sociale', *Les cahiers de droit*, 58(4): 749–87.

Schneider, A. and Ingram, H. (1990) 'Behavioral assumptions of policy tools', *The Journal of Politics*, 52(2): 510–29.

Schneyer, T. (2013) 'The case for proactive management-based regulation to improve professional self-regulation for US lawyers', *Hofstra Law Review*, 42(1): 233.

Scott, W.R. (2008) 'Lords of the dance: Professionals as institutional agents', *Organization Studies*, 29(2): 219–38.

Scott, W.R., Ruef, M., Mendel, P.J. and Caronna, C.A. (2000) *Institutional Change and Health Care Organizations: From Professional Dominance to Managed Care*, Chicago, IL: University of Chicago Press.

Secretaries of State for Health, Wales, Northern Ireland, and Scotland (1989) *Working for Patients*, Cmnd 555, London: HMSO.

Secretary of State for Health (1997) *The New NHS: Modern, Dependable*, London: HMSO.

Secretary of State for Health (1998) *A First Class Service: Quality in the New NHS*, London: HMSO.

Secretary of State for Health (2000) *The NHS Plan: A Plan for Investment, a Plan for Reform*, London: HMSO.

Secretary of State for Health (2004) *The NHS Improvement Plan, CM 6268*, London: TSO.

Secretary of State for Health (2008) *High Quality Care for All: NHS Next Stage Review, Final Report*, Cm 7432, London: HMSO.

Secretary of State for Health (2010) *Equity and Excellence: Liberating the NHS*, London: HMSO.

Secretary of State for Health (2011) *Government Response to the NHS Future Forum Report*, London: Department of Health.

Secretary of State for Health and Social Services (1972) *National Health Service Reorganisation: England*, London: HMSO.

Sehested, K. (2002) 'How new public management reforms challenge the roles of professionals', *International Journal of Public Administration*, 25(12): 1513–37.

Select Committee on the Constitution (2017–19) *The Legislative Process: Preparing Legislation for Parliament*, 4th report (HL 27) 14.

Shaw, E. (2007) *Losing Labour's Soul? New Labour and the Blair Government 1997–2007*, Abingdon: Routledge.

Sheard, S. and Donaldson, L.J. (2006) *The Nation's Doctor: The Role of the Chief Medical Officer 1855–1998*, Oxford: Radcliffe Publishing.

Siddique, H. (2016) 'NHS transformation plans may be used as cover for cuts, says BMA', *The Guardian*, 21 November.

Siebert, S., Martin, G. and Bozic, B. (2016) 'Research into employee trust: Epistemological foundations and paradigmatic boundaries', *Human Resource Management Journal*, 26(3): 269–84.

Sirois, A. (2002a) 'Les médecins veulent casser la loi d'exception', *La Presse*, 2 août.

Sirois, A. (2002b) 'Front commun des médecins contre la loi spéciale' *La Presse*, 12 juillet.

Sirois, A. (2002c) 'Les médecins sont maintenant tenus de divulguer les erreurs médicales', *La Presse*, 8 novembre.

Sirois, A. (2002d) 'Les spécialistes et Québec toujours à couteau tirés', *La Presse*, 26 novembre.

Sirois, A. and Breton, P. (2002) 'Les spécialistes feront une autre journée d'étude en décembre', *La Presse*, 14 novembre.

Smith, D.J. (2002) *The Shipman Inquiry: First Report, Volume One: Death Disguised*, London: HMSO.

Smith, D.J. (2004) *The Shipman Inquiry: Safeguarding Patients: Lessons from the Past – Proposals for the Future* (Fifth report), Cm 6394, London: TSO.

Smith, M.J. (1993) *Pressure, Power and Policy*, London: Harvester Wheatsheaf.

Smith, R. (2003) 'The failures of two contracts', *British Medical Journal*, 326: 1097–8.

Smyth, C., Sylvester, R. and Thomson, A. (2014) 'NHS reforms our worst mistake, Tories admit', *The Times*, 13 October.

Snoddon, T.R. (1998) 'The impact of the CHST on interprovincial redistribution in Canada', *Canadian Public Policy/Analyse de Politiques*, 24(1): 49–70.

Spurgeon, P., Mazelan, P.M. and Barwell, F. (2011) 'Medical engagement: A crucial underpinning to organizational performance', *Health Services Management Research*, 24(3): 114–20.

Starr, P. (1982) *The Social Transformation of American Medicine*, New York, NY: Basic Books.

Strumpf, E., Levesque, J.F., Coyle, N., Hutchison, B., Barnes, M. and Wedel, R.J. (2012) 'Innovative and diverse strategies toward primary health care reform: Lessons learned from the Canadian experience', *The Journal of the American Board of Family Medicine*, 25(Suppl 1): S27–S33.

Stuffco, J. (2013) 'The consensus man', *Medical Post*, 49(1): 29 January.

Suddaby, R. and Greenwood, R. (2009) 'Methodological issues in researching institutional change', in D.A. Buchanan and A. Bryman (eds) *The SAGE Handbook of Organizational Research Methods*, London: SAGE Publications Ltd, pp 177–95.

Suddaby, R. and Viale, T. (2011) 'Professionals and field-level change: Institutional work and the professional project', *Current Sociology*, 59(4): 423–42.

Suddaby, R. and Muzio, D. (2015) 'Theoretical perspectives on the professions', in L. Empson, D. Muzio, J. Broschak and B. Hinings (eds) *The Oxford Handbook of Professional Service Firms*, Oxford: Oxford Handbooks Online, pp 25–47.

Suddaby, R., Cooper, D.J. and Greenwood, R. (2007) 'Transnational regulation of professional services: Governance dynamics of field level organizational change', *Accounting, Organizations and Society*, 32(4–5): 333–62.

Suddaby, R., Gendron, Y. and Lam, H. (2009) 'The organizational context of professionalism in accounting', *Accounting, Organizations and Society*, 34(3–4): 409–27.

Sullivan, P. (1990) 'Debate heated, but OMA backs deferral of court challenge', *Canadian Medical Association Journal*, 143(1): 47–8.

Swedberg, R. (2005) 'Can there be a sociological concept of interest?', *Theory and Society*, 34(4): 359–90.

Sylvain, M. (2010) 'Ontario hospitals mull MD assessment system', *Medical Post*, 46(17): 32–3.

Sylvain, M. (2011a) 'OMA readying master-agreement negotiations strategy', *Medical Post*, 47(9): 40.

Sylvain, M. (2011b) 'Former negotiator takes helm of Ontario Medical Association', *Medical Post*, 47(9): 4.

Taylor, M. (2009) *Health Insurance and Canadian Public Policy: The Seven Decisions that Created the Health Insurance System and Their Outomes*, Montréal, QC: McGill-Queen's University Press. Available at: www.jstor. org/stable/j.ctt80w3s.7?refreqid=excelsior%3A7b128c836bb09c4914531 18ff0882303&seq=68#metadata_info_tab_contents

Tenszen, M. (1991) 'Doctors okay 6-year deal that pits cap on billing', *Toronto Star*, 28 May.

Thatcher, M. (1980) 'The lady's not for turning', Conservative Party Conference.

Thatcher, M. (1993) *The Downing Street Years*, London: HarperCollins.

Timmins, N. (1995) *The Five Giants: A Biography of the Welfare State*, London: Fontana Books.

Timmins, N. (2008) 'NHS urged to share market system', *Financial Times*, 7 July.

Timmins, N. (2010) 'Doctors attack business involvement in the NHS', *Financial Times*, 12 February.

Timmins, N. (2012) *Never Again? The Story of the Health and Social Care Act 2012*, London: The King's Fund.

Titmuss, R. (1958) *Essays on the Welfare State*, Cambridge: Polity Press.

Tyler, T.R. (2011) *Why People Cooperate: The Role Of Social Motivations*, Princeton, NJ: Princeton University Press.

Torfing, J. (2005) 'Governance network theory: Towards a second generation', *European Political Science*, 4(3): 305–15.

Toronto Star (1966a) 'Anti-Medicare pledge by 4,500 doctors makes Dymond "ashamed"', 18 February.

Toronto Star (1966b) 'OMSIP does not qualify for federal aid: MacEachen', 6 June.

Toronto Star (1966c) 'MDs' pamphlets in waiting rooms aimed at OMSIP', 2 August.

Toronto Star (1967) 'Doctors said "irresponsible" over their fee increase', 11 April.

Toronto Star (1968) 'Ontario doctors want raise of 10% in some fees', 11 November.

Toronto Star (1971a) 'New law forbids double billing by Ontario doctors', 25 June.

Toronto Star (1971b) (OMA) 'An open letter to the citizens of Ontario', 7 July.

Toronto Star (1972) 'More health clinics planned', 11 May.

Toronto Star (1980) 'How OMA, Ontario settle fees', 7 June.

Toronto Star (1989) 'Cap on fees denounced by former OMA head', 13 April.

Torstendahl, R. (2005) 'The need for a definition of "profession"', *Current Sociology*, 53(6): 947–51.

Tsoukas, H. and Chia, R. (2002) 'On organizational becoming: Rethinking organizational change', *Organization Science*, 13(5): 567–82.

Tuohy, C.H. (1999) *Accidental Logics: The Dynamics of Change in the Health Care Arena in the United States, Britain, and Canada*, Oxford: Oxford University Press.

Tuohy, C.H. (2012) 'Reform and the politics of hybridization in mature health care states', *Journal of Health Politics, Policy and Law*, 37(4): 611–32.

Tuohy, C.H. (2018). *Remaking Policy: Scale, Pace, and Political Strategy in Health Care Reform* (Vol 54), Toronto, ON: University of Toronto Press.

Tuohy, C.J. (1988) 'Medicine and the state in Canada: The extra-billing issue in perspective', *Canadian Journal of Political Science Revue canadienne de science politique*, 267–96.

Turner, B.S. (1995) *Medical Power and Social Knowledge*, London: SAGE Publications Ltd.

Usher S., Denis, J-L., Côté-Boileau, E., Préval, J., Baker, G.R. and Chreim S. (2020) 'What does it mean to have quality drive healthcare reforms? Ontario's experience' at the 12th Organisational Behaviour in Health Care (OBHC) Conference, Manchester, UK, April.

van Gestel, N., Denis, J.L., Ferlie, E. and McDermott, A.M. (2018) 'Explaining the policy process underpinning public sector reform: The role of ideas, institutions, and timing', *Perspectives on Public Management and Governance*, 1(2): 87–101.

Vogel, L. (2010) 'Ontario Hospital Association proposes to scuttle privileges model for doctors', *Canadian Medical Association Journal*, 13 July.

Vollant S. and Senikas A. (2002) 'Urgences: des solutions durables', *La Presse*, 11 July, A 14.

Waldegrave, W. (1991) 'William Waldegrave: Thinking on the NHS. Interview by Richard Smith', *British Medical Journal*, 302: 636.

Walker, P., Allegretti, A. and Quinn, B. (2021) 'Anger grows at offer of 1% pay rise for NHS staff', *The Guardian*, 5 March.

Walkom, T. (1993) 'Physicians healed themselves quite nicely', *Toronto Star*, 9 August.

Wansbrough, G. (1998) 'NP's privileges extended', *Medical Post*, 34(9): 109.

Ward, B. (1983) 'Begin ready to get tough on Medicare', *Toronto Star*, 26 July.

Waring, J. and Bevir, M. (2017) 'Decentring health policy: Traditions, narratives, dilemmas', in M. Bevir and J. Waring (eds) *Decentring Health Policy*, Abingdon: Routledge, pp 13–28.

Waring, J., Latif, A., Boyd, M., Barber, N. and Elliott, R. (2016) 'Pastoral power in the community pharmacy: A Foucauldian analysis of services to promote patient adherence to new medicine use', *Social Science & Medicine*, 148: 123–30.

Webster, C. (1988) *The Health Services Since the War: The National Health Service before 1957* (Vol 1), London: HM Stationery Office.

Weiers, M. (1979) 'Frustration over OHIP regulations builds among doctors', *Toronto Star*, 24 April.

Wilensky, H.L. (1964) 'The professionalization of everyone?', *American Journal of Sociology*, 70(2): 137–58.

Women and Equalities Committee (2020) *Unequal Impact? Coronavirus and BAME People*, London: House of Commons.

Wu, X., Ramesh, M., and Howlett, M. (2015) 'Policy capacity: A conceptual framework for understanding policy competences and capabilities', *Policy and Society*, 34(3–4): 165–71.

Wuldart, Y. (1966) 'Bien réfléchir avant d'instaurer l'assurance-maladie', *La Presse*, 4 janvier.

Wyman, M. (1989) 'It's a sad day for medicine in Ontario', *Canadian Medical Association Journal*, 140: 202–3.

Yiu, V., Belanger, F. and Todd, K. (2019) 'Alberta's Strategic Clinical Networks: Enabling health system innovation and improvement', *Canadian Medical Association Journals*, 191(Suppl): S1–S3.

Zietsma, C., Groenewegen, P., Logue, D.M. and Hinings, C.R. (2017) 'Field or fields? Building the scaffolding for cumulation of research on institutional fields', *Academy of Management Annals*, 11(1): 391–450.

Index

References to figures appear in *italic* type.
References to endnotes show both the
page number and the note number (94n7).